Praise for Drunk Yoga®

(*Real* quotes said by *real* people about *real* Drunk Yoga® classes taught by the *real* Eli Walker.)

"So *not* what I expected in the best way possible."

"It's like the best drinking game . . . ever."

"I was finally able to bring my boyfriend to yoga. He *loved* it. Cheers!"

"The most fun I've ever had in a yoga class."

"I have never laughed so hard in a yoga class in my entire life."

"Eli is an inspiration—she's changed the way I think about yoga."

"I've never seen so many strangers come together in one room and then compliment one another so much."

"Thank you, Eli, for enriching our lives."

"Eli's Drunk Yoga® class reminds me why I love yoga."

"It was my first yoga class . . . now I get it."

"I'm not flexible, but in Drunk Yoga® I forgot. Thanks for making something scary to me so much fun."

"I don't even drink and I totally love Drunk Yoga®."

"For a nondrinker, this is totally intoxicating in all the best ways."

"We had an absolutely terrific Sunday Funday! Girls' day, beautiful weather, met fun people, and enjoyed ourselves all around! Also, I don't do yoga, so I found it totally awesome doing basic moves, and the wine made it fun, too. Our class was on a yacht, so we were totally having a good time!"

"At first, I thought it was so dumb . . . so *not* what yoga is. Took a chance, went—I see now that it's for real."

"Eli is a real yoga teacher. She knows exactly what she's doing. Everyone should try this class."

"I brought a man to Drunk Yoga® who had never taken any kind of yoga class before. Before it was over, he said, 'We need to do this again!'"

"Best bachelorette party *ever*."

"Now that I'm thirty, I feel like I can't *just* drink on the weekends. I need to work out, too, so Drunk Yoga® is perfect for me."

"I don't know if Drunk Yoga® makes me more flexible, but once class started, I sort of forgot to care."

"Eli Walker is a visionary."

Drunk Yoga®

50 WINE & YOGA POSES TO LIFT YOUR SPIRIT(S)

Eli Walker

ILLUSTRATIONS BY JUSTIN PETTIT

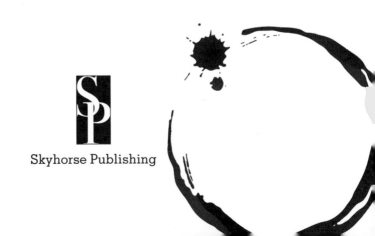

Skyhorse Publishing

Skyhorse Publishing books may be purchased in bulk at special discounts for sales promotion, corporate gifts, fund-raising, or educational purposes. Special editions can also be created to specifications. For details, contact the Special Sales Department, Skyhorse Publishing, 307 West 36th Street, 11th Floor, New York, NY 10018 or info@skyhorsepublishing.com.

Skyhorse® and Skyhorse Publishing® are registered trademarks of Skyhorse Publishing, Inc.®, a Delaware corporation. Visit our website at www.skyhorsepublishing.com.

10 9 8 7 6 5 4 3 2 1

Library of Congress Cataloging-in-Publication Data is available on file.

Cover design by Mona Lin
Cover photographs by Meagan Stevenson
Cover illustrations by Justin Pettit

Print ISBN: 978-1-5107-4082-2
Ebook ISBN: 978-1-5107-4083-9

Printed in China

To Mom, Dad, and Michael.
Thanks for always allowing me to force you to listen to my stories.

And to New York City and Bali, and the ~~humans~~ angels
living in them who helped me get here.

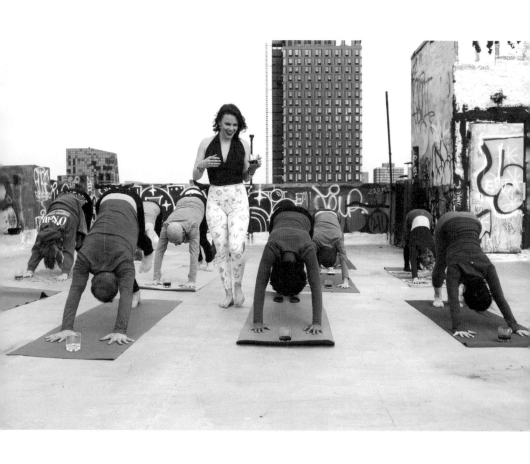

TABLE OF CONTENTS

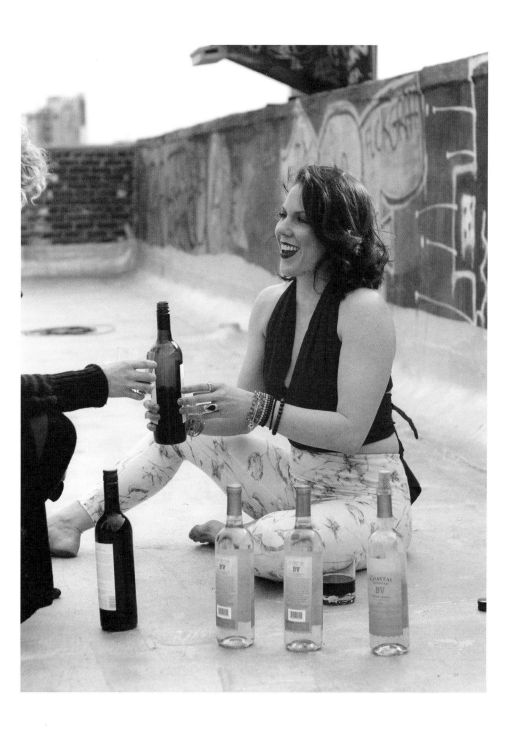

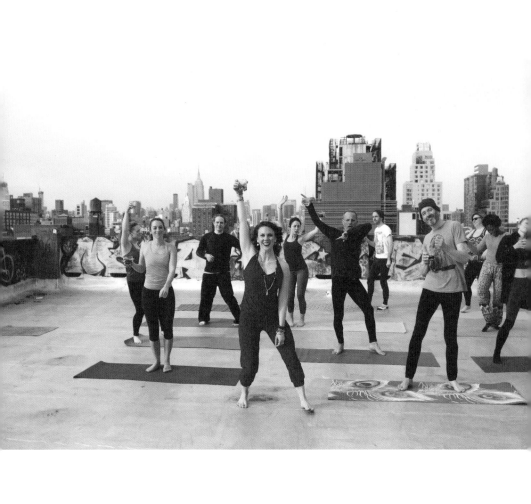

INTRODUCTION

I had no intention of making such a splash with Drunk Yoga®. I thought of the idea one night while I was out at a bar called Grey Lady in Lower Manhattan, where I used to work right after college.

I was catching up with a friend, who was the coowner of the bar. I told him that I'm a yoga teacher now. He said, "I need yoga, I can't touch my toes." Then, he immediately proceeded to touch his toes. "Oh," he said, surprised. "I guess I can touch my toes when I'm drunk." (Cue light bulb moment.) With excitement, I blurted, "Well then, let's just do Drunk Yoga®! I'll teach a class in the bar's back room for beginners. It'll be fun." He loved the idea and responded, "Sure! What should we call it? 'Tipsy Yoga'?" Definitively, as if the gods above had just granted me permission from the Drunk Yoga® heavens, I said, "No. I want to call it 'Drunk Yoga®.'"

The first few classes were empty. I planned to scrap the idea, as I was in the midst of preparing to teach a (sober) yoga retreat in Bali. But, in one last-ditch effort to pull in a crowd, I reached out to my friend who wrote for *Gothamist*, dragged her to a class, and begged her to write about it.

Soon after her article was published, news outlet after news outlet across the globe wrote about the story. "Eli Walker's Drunk Yoga® class is the latest trend in NYC . . .," they said— "New York City's Eli Walker offers 'liquid courage' to beginner yogis to welcome them to the practice. . . . " Fans of the class were ecstatic, and reservations began *pouring* in as Drunk Yoga® went viral overnight.

I quickly realized that through the Drunk Yoga® phenomenon, I had touched on something much greater than our culture's love for mixing alcohol with . . . everything. I realized there is a societal thirst for a breaking away from what has become an exclusive yoga elite, reserved for the wealthy and the flexible. And although the polarizing name of my new endeavor hit a nerve with some yoga purists, I feel pleased to be igniting a conversation that dares to deconstruct the essence of what it truly means to "do yoga."

You see, I've spent many years mildly obsessed with developing ways to integrate performance with yoga to offer unconventional ways of teaching people the art of joy through self-empowerment. Drunk Yoga®, so far, has been the most effective twist. It has the power to spread yoga to the uninitiated through accessible means: wine and socializing.

Furthermore, there comes a point in a yoga teacher's career when the teaching moves beyond the instruction of the poses and into the realm of what it means to be a radiant human being. Yoga to me is much like performance. It's about learning to develop a relationship to one's own body in time and space, for the ultimate purpose of cultivating personal happiness. And, when we have techniques to uplift ourselves, we can work better in community to uplift one another. Drunk Yoga® is about just that: finding levity in the communal.

Wine is, inarguably, a tool to bring people together. Add a little wine to any situation, and it turns into a celebration. And in Drunk Yoga®, we're celebrating the soul and nurturing it through the ritual of a "happy hour." The ritualization of a "happy hour" through the structure of a yoga class is like the theater of communal celebration. The result is a magical breakdown of barriers through socializing to expose our inherent playfulness.

So, in summary: (clears throat) I use the word "Drunk" suggestively and sarcastically. It's not "descriptive," as my trademark lawyer will have you note. Drunk Yoga® combines expressive yoga sans pressure to be perfect, painted with the theater of happy hour (socializing) and risk-taking (Drunk Yoga® is shamelessly subversive, have you heard?) in such a beautiful blend (like Grenache, you know?) that opens the space for collaborative joy! (It's fun as f#ck,* and happiness *is* health.)

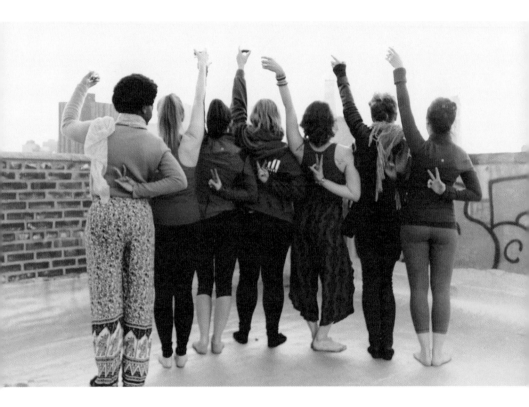

---

* My editor doesn't want me to swear.

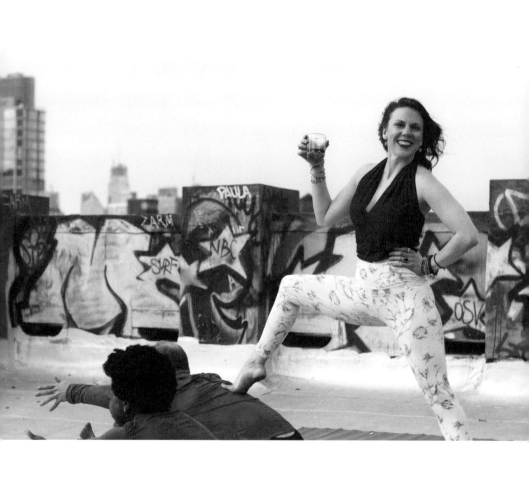

Wine Not?

Because everything happens for a Riesling. Making "pour" decisions is part of being human. #loveyourself. (Whew. I've been *dying* for a reason to use those puns since I started Drunk Yoga®. Thanks for letting me get that out of my system before we dive in.)

Yoga can be as lightheartedly fun or as deeply personal as you make it. And it should be both. Yoga means "unity." It is the awakened experience of your life. I've seen people get turned off by yoga, or develop an aversion to it, because, for many, it can appear too regimented and commercialized, as it is widely marketed for the already fit and flexible.

But here's the thing: there are ba*jillions* of ways to yoga. Just *one* way is to do it with wine in your hand in the back of a bar. And lucky for you, here's a book about it!

Don't drink alcohol but still want to join in on the fun? No problem! Drunk Yoga® is about uplifting spirits through community, and if for you that means lifting a glass of coconut water, kombucha, or coffee, more power to you! (But be careful with the coffee, yeah? The only thing more dangerous than wine and yoga is scalding hot coffee and yoga, in my bona fide professional opinion.)

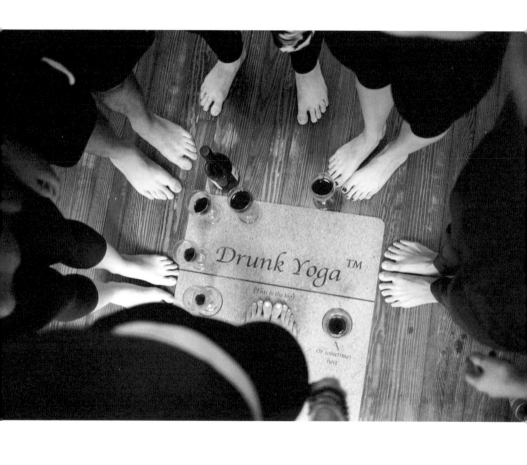

Drunk Yoga® Class Rules

1. If you lose your balance, take a sip.

2. No spilling . . . and when you *do* spill your wine and you *need* to refill your glass, you must pour while doing a yoga pose. (Tree pose is the Drunk Yoga® favorite; see page 61.)

3. If you spill wine on your neighbor's mat, you must give him or her a compliment.

4. If you spill on your own mat, you must give *yourself* a compliment.

5. If you take a sip without being instructed to do so during class, you must give *the teacher* a compliment.

6. If you say something self-deprecating, you need to high-five your neighbor and say, "I'm awesome!"

7. If you mix up your "left" and "right" appendages, you must tell the class something that you're grateful for.

8. If you drop your (reusable/biodegradable) straw, you have to make up the next yoga pose for the class.

9. The Drunk Yoga® teacher reserves the right to make up new rules whenever the "spirit(s)" move(s) her/him.

10. Leave the classroom happier than when you entered.

SOBER YOGA: CHILD'S POSE
SANSKRIT: *BALASANA*

Drunk Yoga®: Bottle-asana

This wine was trapped in a bottle, but don't worry—we rescued it.

Spread your knees as wide as the mat and reach your butt bones to your heels. Reach your arms out long in front of you. Rest your forehead on the mat. Close your eyes.

This is your excuse to be lazy. I mean, this is a resting pose.

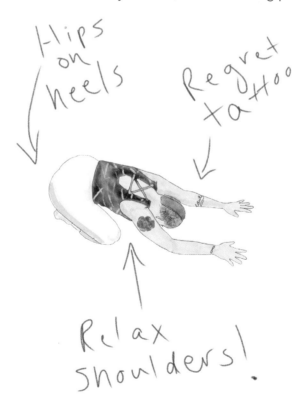

Hips on heels

Regret tattoo

Relax shoulders!

Drunk Yoga®: I'll-do-more-o'-that-saw-asana

Goal: to create an equilateral triangle with your body (three 60-degree angles) and truly embody the archetype of a dog stretching.

Hands at the top of the mat, shoulder-width apart.

Feet hips-width apart, driving heels into the mat.

Knees soft and buttock bones reaching up.

Draw the shoulder blades back and down and keep the vision between the knees.

Sense that your heart is peeking forward to give your back a slight bend.

You may feel like you're using muscles you didn't even know you had in this pose. Your arms and legs might start to shake, and your hands might start to slip on the mat.

Just keep your cool. If your dog can do this, you can do it, too.

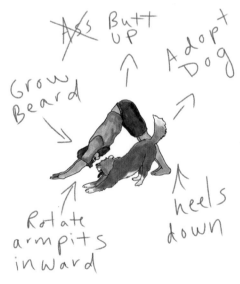

Ass Butt UP

Grow Beard

Adopt Dog

Rotate armpits inward

heels down

*Drunk Yoga®: On-rocks-ana**

Stand at the top of your mat with your feet parallel and hips-width distance apart.

Stack your shoulders directly over your hips, your hips over your knees, and your knees over your ankles.

Your face, shoulders, and booty**
are relaxed.

Bring your wine to heart center to
begin.

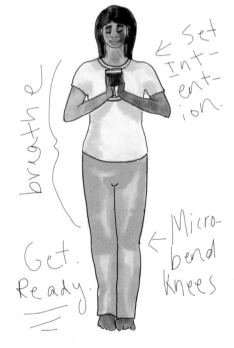

breathe

← *Set Intention.*

Get. Ready.

← *Micro-bend knees*

---

* If you're the kind of person who puts ice in their wineglass. #nojudgment #actually #yeah #alittlejudgment

** #shakeshakeshake

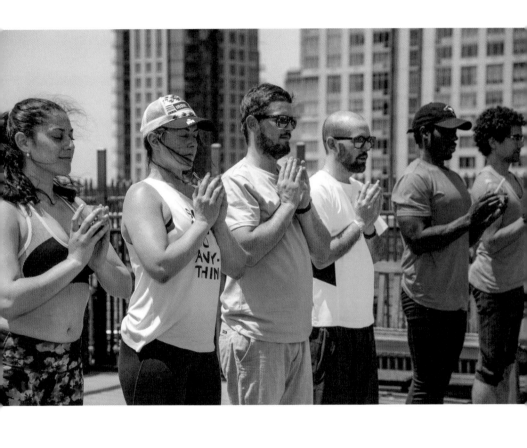

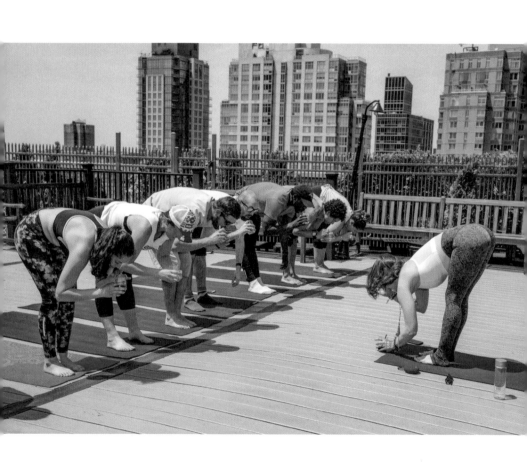

SOBER YOGA: STANDING FORWARD BEND
SANSKRIT: UTTANASANA
Drunk Yoga®: Oops-tanasana*

From a standing position with wine in hand and feet hips-width apart, hinge from the hips and fold yourself in half.

(This is the point at which you'll probably spill.)

The buttock bones rise as you distribute your weight equally between the balls of each foot and the heels of each foot.

Set your glass of wine down in front of your mat and place your palms outside of your feet.

While you're down there, maybe grab a towel, a sock, or someone else's tee shirt (with consent) and wipe up the splash you just made, ya big splasher!

. . . And then give yourself a compliment, because we all make mistakes, and those are the rules.

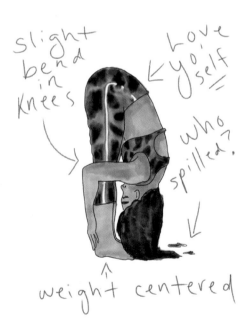

slight bend in knees

Love yourself

who spilled.

weight centered

---

* You're probably going to spill your wine in this pose.

Drunk Yoga®: (Salamba) Beaujolais-ana

Begin lying on your front. Prop yourself up on your forearms and draw the shoulder blades back and down. Press the tops of your feet and your hips down onto the mat as you lengthen your neck and throat. Make an effort to lengthen your lower back, so as not to compress it.

For extra credit, lean your head forward and take a sip *with no hands*.

Nice job! High five! So proud. I have stickers, do you want one?

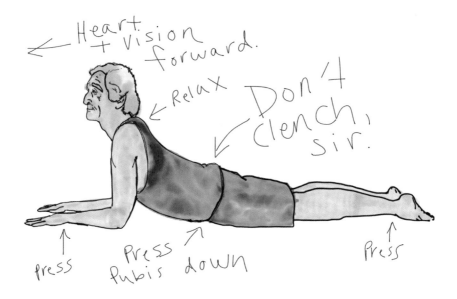

← Heart + vision forward.
← Relax
Don't clench, sir.
press
Press Pubis down
Press

Drunk Yoga®: Come-back-asana*

From downward-facing dog, bring your shoulders over your wrists so that your arms are perpendicular to the ground, forming a 90-degree angle.

Draw your navel in toward your spine to engage your abdominal muscles and engage your legs as you actively reach your heels backward.

Spread your fingers wide and distribute your weight equally between the balls of your feet and your knuckles.

Pretend your body is aligned and sturdy like a long wooden board. Or something else that's long, hard, and sturdy . . .

. . . like a marble countertop, or a bookshelf that's not from IKEA.

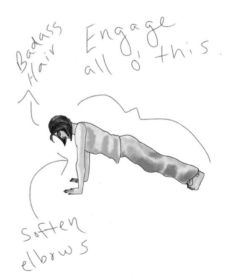

Badass Hair

Engage all o' this.

Soften elbrws

---

* What you somberly mutter into your empty wineglass when you realize that you already drank it all.

Drunk Yoga®: Beaujolais-ana

In preparation, place the glass at the top of the mat with a (reusable/biodegradable) straw.

Lying facedown on your mat, squeeze your legs together and press the tops of your feet on the ground as you use the muscles of your lower back to lift your chest. Your elbows are bent and knitted in close to the rib cage, and your palms lift a couple of inches off the ground.

Without using your hands, take a sip from a (reusable/biodegradable) straw.

. . . Because fun.

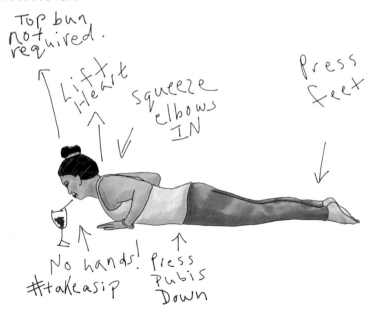

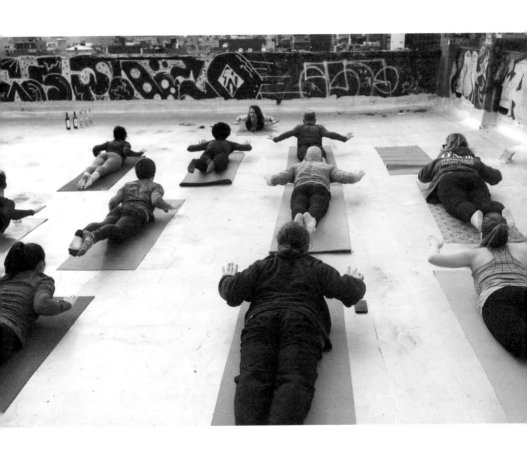

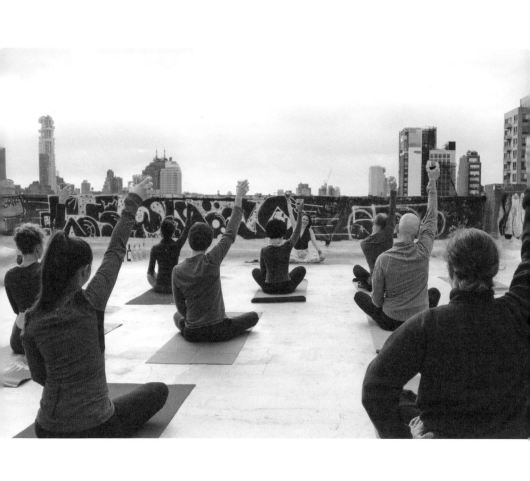

WHAT YOGA IS

"A technology for happiness."—Nayaswami Gyandev McCord

"Yoga is how you stop time from doing you in."—Nevine Michaan

"Yoga got me through the Civil War."—Abraham Lincoln

"Yoga is the removal of the fluctuations of the mind."—Patanjali

"A cult!"—your Great-Aunt Mary

"Yoga means having an easeful body, a peaceful mind, and a useful life."—Swami Satchidananda

"Yoga is for crazies."—Republicans

"We're not crazy! We're just living our truth."—Democrats

"Me, obvs."—God

"Yoga is a tool to help you develop a better relationship to yourself, for the purpose of having a more joyful life journey. Yoga is a universal practice of unifying the mind, body, and spirit; it's a celebration of what it means to be alive through a moving meditation that cultivates graciousness through spaciousness . . . sometimes by yourself. Sometimes with others. Sometimes with water.* Maybe in a bar with your best friends while singing to Beyoncé and/or by yourself at home in your underwear listening to Disney musical soundtracks on full blast."—Me (for whatever the heck that's worth) #drunkyoga #liftyourspirits #liveyourbestlife

---

* And sometimes with wine.

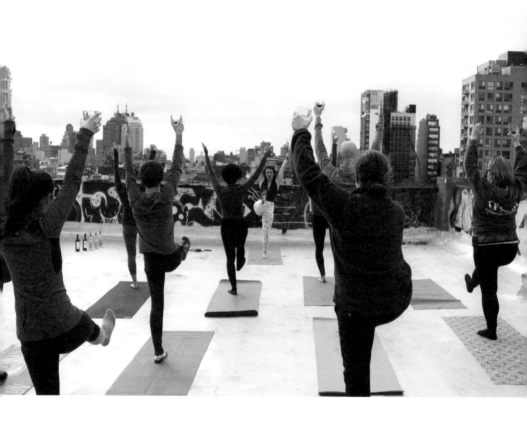

WHAT YOGA ISN'T, IN VERSE

Yoga is not just for hippies or for yuppies.
It is more than imitating downward-facing puppies.
Yoga isn't an excuse to show us your abs on Instagram.
And it's more than sitting cross-legged, pondering, "Who I am."
Yoga is not a style of pants.
It's not about marching like an army of ants.
Yoga is much, much more than gymnastics.
Oh yes, you see, it's much more fantastic.
Yoga is not reserved for the wealthy or the healthy.
And it's *certainly* not just for old levitating Indian men—boy,
they're stealthy.
The magic of yoga reaches farther than the eyes.
But please don't assume that all yogis are spies.
In fact, my good friends, yogis are just like you and me.
They laugh, they cry, they yawn, they pee.

Yoga gives you more than phenomenal @sses.
And best of all, it's free! (. . . Except when it's $20 per classes.)
Yoga was made for land and for sea.
Yes yogaaaa was made for you and meeee.
No but seriously, it's a universal practice.
It's about more than making skinny girls' joints look elastic.
Be you big, be you small,
Be you short, be you tall,
Yoga brings joy to any and all.
"How does it do this?" . . . With a raised eyebrow, you ask.
Try it for yourself, if you're up to the task!
Only through your own personal experience can you see
That unifying breath, body, mind, and spirit is key.
Yes, uh-huh, for *sure*, yup, *totally*, indeed.
Yogaaaa was made for you and meeeee.
(. . . No, but, seriously, you should try it.)

*Drunk Yoga®: Marge-arch-your-as(s)-ana**

On your hands and knees, creating 90-degree angles with the arms and legs, press down into the ground with the tops of your feet as you bring weight into the knuckles of your first fingers to relieve pressure from your wrists.

Inhale as you draw your navel in toward your spine and round your back. Tuck your chin into your chest, and your pelvis in and up.

Basically, you're embodying the archetype of a cat that is jumping five feet in the air from fright after it "accidentally" knocked your wineglass off the counter. #notcool

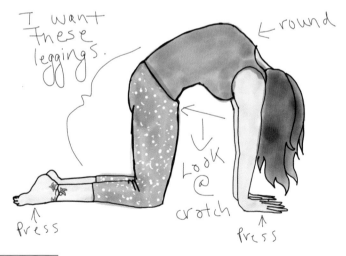

I want these leggings.

← round

Look @ crotch

Press

Press

---

* When your cat's name is "Marge."

SOBER YOGA: YOGI PUSH-UP
SANSKRIT: CHATURANGA

Drunk Yoga®: Shot-a-ranga*

Begin in a plank position. As you exhale, slowly bend your elbows to 90-degree angles, as if to do a push-up. Hold for a breath, and take a sip. Be sure to keep your elbows close to the rib cage, and your core engaged.

Note: More advanced yogis may push themselves back to plank on the next inhale, post-sip. Beginner yogis may find it best to dramatically collapse onto their bellies for a brief moment. Additional sip of liquid courage is optional.

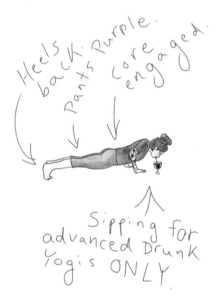

Heels back.
Purple pants.
core engaged.

Sipping for advanced Drunk Yogis ONLY

---

* Sorry, misleading pun. No liquor shots allowed in Drunk Yoga®—only champagne shots! (For highly scientific purposes. And by "scientific," I mean "insurance.")

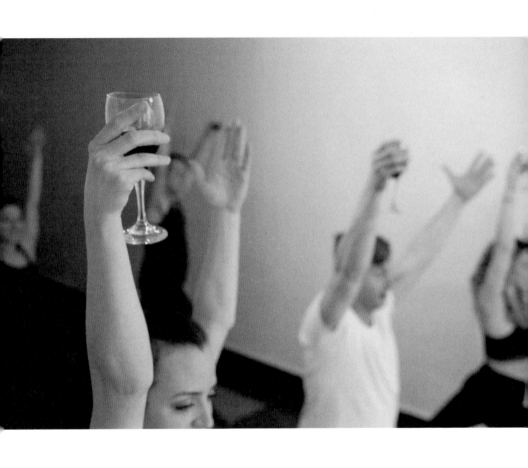

Sober Yoga: "Flow"
Sanskrit: *Vinyasa*
Drunk Yoga®: Vinoyasa

Place your glass of wine in the center of the top of your yoga mat. Come into a plank pose.

Inhale to prepare. As you exhale, bring just your knees, chest, and chin to the mat *or* exhale into shot-a-ranga. As you inhale, slide forward for baby cobra and take a sip. Exhale, tuck your toes, and lift your body back into a downward-facing dog.

Advanced variation—use aforementioned straw to sip mid-shot-a-ranga.

Offer for stickers is still on the table.

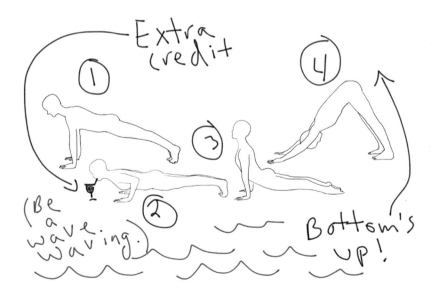

Extra credit

(Be waving.)

Bottom's up!

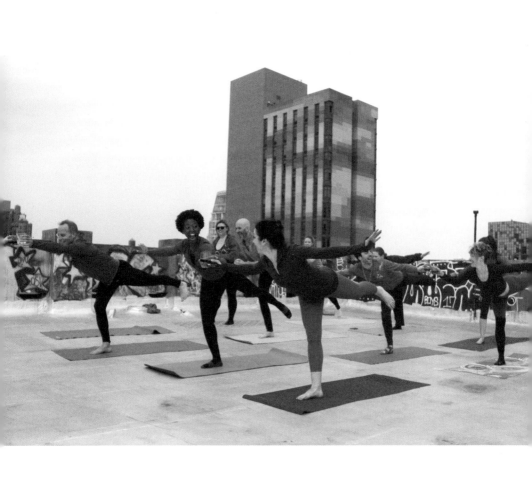

10 Common Side Effects of Yoga

1. Inexplicable contentment

2. That feeling of, like, "Psh, yeah! I *got* this."

3. May suddenly forget what you were just worried about

4. An overwhelming appreciation for friends and family

5. A love of "self"

6. Compassion for your body

7. Compassion for mankind

8. Compassion for animal-kind

9. Overwhelming craving for green juice. #sorrynotsorry

10. A great night of sleep

11. Clearer mind for conscious decision ma-. . . oh wait, sorry, I said "10." Never mind. Forget it.

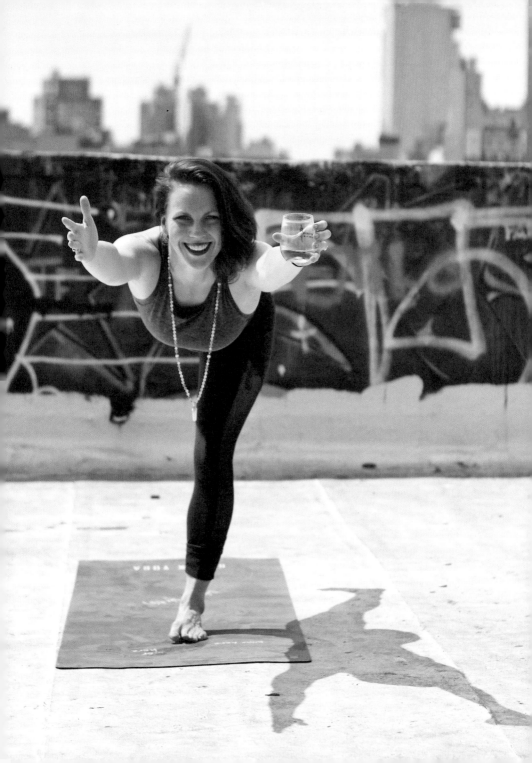

A Thoroughly Comprehensive List . . .

(. . . of 25 activities that are pretty great sober,
but slightly more enjoyable with a glass of wine)

1. (Literally everything.)

2. See #1

3. See #1

4. See #1

5. See #1

6. See #1

7. See #1

8. See #1

9. See #1

10. See #1

11. See #1

12. See #1

13. See #1

14. See #1

15. See #1

16. See #1

17. See #1

18. See #1

19. See #1

20. See #1

21. See #1

22. See #1

23. See #1

24. See #1

25. See #1

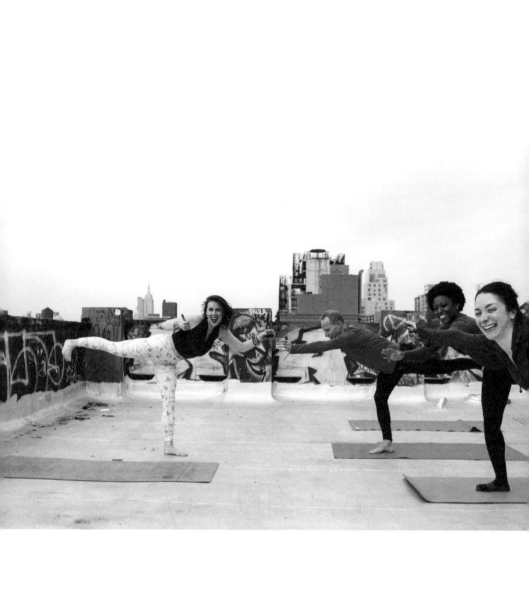

BREAKING (WIND) NEWS: PRO TIPS ON FARTING*

If you fart during yoga, you're doing it right.

Still, much like any undesirable bodily function, just because it's "natural" doesn't mean it's "cute." Nobody wants to be *that* yogi in class who totally lets one rip in plow pose, be it a fart *or*, God forbid, a queef.**

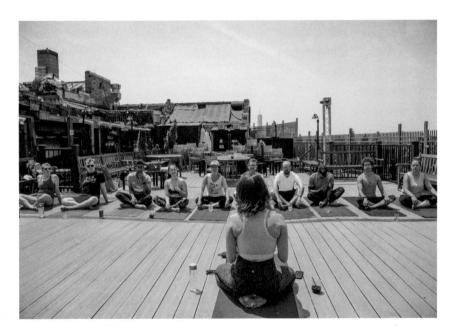

---

* Except the teacher. We don't fart.
** Confused? Google it. I'm not explaining it here—this book is rated G. (well, PG. Okay fine, PG-13.)

Drunk Yoga®: Moo-mo-sana

For best results, practice with mimosas.

Typically done in conjunction with cat pose. So, when you are finished embodying the archetype of a terrified cat, exhale and allow your torso to curve as you drop your belly and extend your heart and throat, and gaze upward. Don't forget to stick your butt* out. And, no need to actually "moo" here, people. This is *Drunk Yoga®*, not *LSD* yoga.

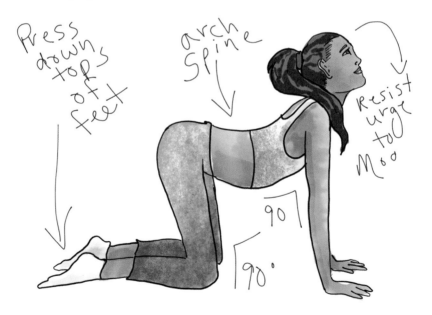

---

* @$$

Drunk Yoga®: Croissant Pose

Pretend you're in France and eating a croissant with wine. (Is that a thing?)

From downward-facing dog, move your right leg forward and place your right foot inside your right hand.

Gently place your left knee on the mat and press the top of your left foot down to relieve excess pressure from your left knee.

Make sure that your right knee is directly over your right ankle, and as you're ready, lean your hips forward and raise your arms up so that your fingers are reaching skyward and your upper arms are in line with your ears.

If you didn't bring your wine with you, tough luck. If you did, take a sip.

As you're ready, bring your arms (and wine) down, move into downward-facing dog or vinoyasa, and repeat this pose on the left.

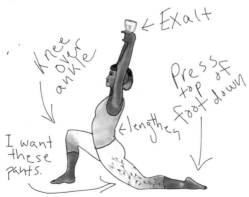

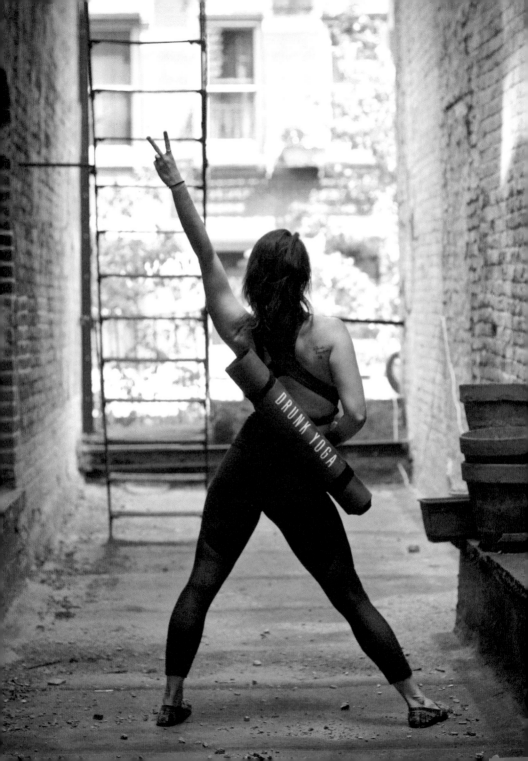

FIND THE BUDDHA,
KILL THE BUDDHA

"If you meet the Buddha, kill him."
—Zen Master Linji

Not literally, obviously.

On the path to enlightenment, through study, meditation, yoga, and prayer, you will meet many figures who will tell you that they know all of the answers. They will tell you what is "wrong" with you, and how they can fix you. And you may surrender your power to them out of respect and humility, hoping with best intentions to evolve.

This proverb advises that as soon as you "meet the Buddha," or rather, "see enlightenment," your conception is wrong, and you must destroy whatever image you see and continue on your own journey.

Not to get all "yoga teacher" on you here, but I want to take a moment to pause from my puns and tell you that *you* are your own best teacher. As you tread your spiritual path, you ought to learn from as many instructors, sages, wise old men, wise young men, and even *wiser* women.

Your life is yours to live, and your identity is yours to claim. To surrender your power to a self-proclaimed guru in the name of spiritual devotion is disrespectful to the very existence you've earned by being alive in a body. The best way to honor your spirit is to let go of any idea that you are "doing life wrong," while others are "doing it right." You are in exactly the right place, at exactly the right time, under exactly the right circumstances. (Otherwise, you would be somewhere else, and someone else, entirely, amirite?)

Drunk Yoga®: Merlot-asana

Separate your feet so your heels are directly underneath your shoulders.

Turn each foot out to a 45-degree angle. Bring your wine to heart center as you use your elbows to gently separate your knees.

Breathe deeply into your lower back, belly, and hips.

Relax your shoulders and take a sip.

For best results, practice pose with merlot.

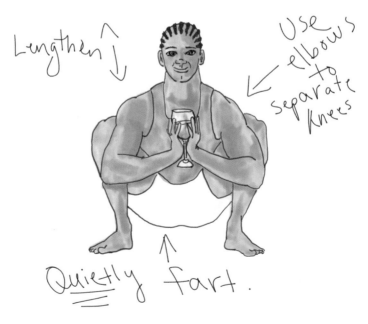

SOBER YOGA: WARRIOR 1
SANSKRIT: *VIRABHADRASANA* 1

Drunk Yoga®: Vino-bad@$$-ana 1

From downward-facing dog, bring your right foot forward and place it next to the inside of your right hand. Spin your left heel down so that your entire left foot is situated at a 45-degree angle, with your toes facing toward 10 o'clock. With square hips, grab ahold of your wineglass with your right hand and slowly come up. Your arms are straight and in line with your ears. Your shoulders are stacked over your hips and rotated inward, while your gaze is forward. Your right knee is directly over your right ankle, forming a stable 90-degree angle in your joint. Your glass of wine remains steady, and you're not spilling it, because you're a total bad@$$ and you've got this.

After about five cycles of breath, lower down with control.

Advanced Drunk Yogis can make a point of dramatically lowering down in slow motion while taking a sip of wine. (Beginners can take a sip sans the slow-motion bit, unless it happens naturally . . . then, in that case, just go with it.)

Place your glass outside your right foot and step back into downward-facing dog, or take a vinoyasa.

Repeat this pose with your left leg forward.

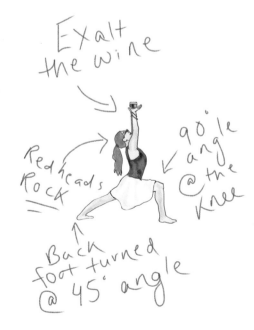

Exalt the wine

Red heads Rock

90° angle @ the knee

Back foot turned @ 45° angle

Drunk Yoga®: *Vino-bad@$$-ana 2*

The same as Vino-bad@$$-ana 1, except completely different.

From downward-facing dog, bring your right foot forward and place it next to the inside of your right hand. Spin your left heel down so that your entire left foot is situated at a 90-degree angle, with your toes and hips facing the left-side wall. Grab ahold of your wineglass with your right hand and slowly come up. Your arms are straight and parallel to the ground. Your shoulders are relaxed and stacked directly over your hips. Your gaze is forward, just beyond your wine. You may also gaze directly at the wine, if this provides you with incentive.

Once again, your right knee is directly above your right ankle, forming a stable 90-degree angle at the joint. The glass of wine remains steady, and you're not spilling it, because, as established in vino-bad@$$-ana 1, you're a total bad@$$ and you've got this.

After about five cycles of breath, lower your arms with control.

Advanced Drunk Yogis can once again make a point of dramatically lowering down in slow motion while taking a sip of wine. (Beginners can take a sip sans the slow-motion bit.)

Place the glass outside your right foot and step back into downward-facing dog, or take a vinoyasa. Repeat this pose with your left leg forward.

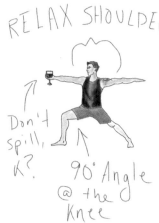

RELAX SHOULDE

Don't spill, k?

90° Angle @ the Knee

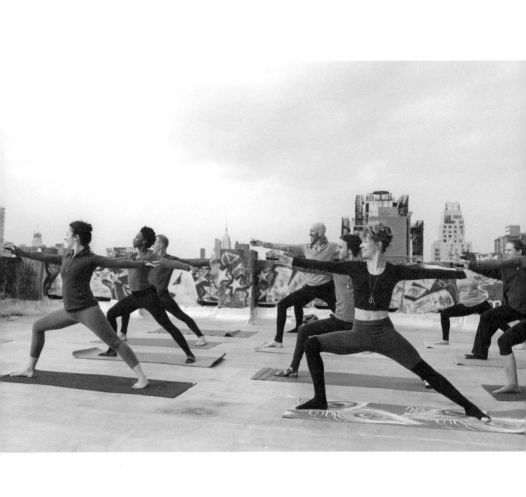

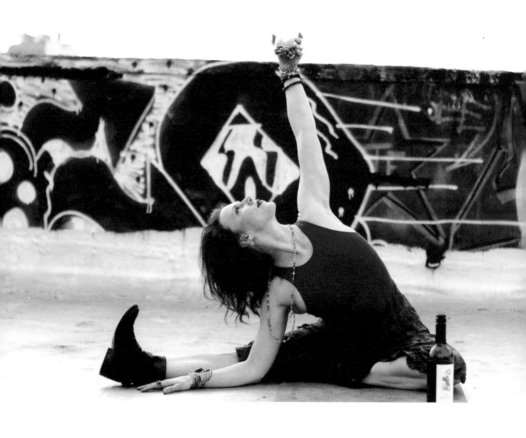

My First Time

Who doesn't remember their first time? Usually sweaty, always messy, and at times painful—for some more than others. The experience opens parts of your body that you didn't even know you had. And once you try it, you'll never be the same again.

Indeed, my first time trying yoga was a real game changer.

My arms were shaking and my palms were sweaty. The yoga teacher came up to me, as I was clearly doing downward-facing dog pose incorrectly—compensating in all the wrong ways with all the wrong body parts. She crouched down in that annoyingly Zen yoga teacher way and whispered, "You need to bring your arms in line with your ears." I whispered back, slightly more aggressively than she did (and by slightly, I mean significantly), "I understand what I'm *supposed* to do, I just can't *do* it." She smiled that infuriatingly serene yoga teacher smile and said, "It'll get easier." She walked—nay, *floated*—away, as I rolled my eyes and thought, *Bull.*

Cut to many years later, obviously, I got a handle on my attitude, because I've been a professional yoga teacher for several years, teaching all over the world. Now *I* get to *float* across yoga studio slash bar floors while barefoot and condescendingly whisper in students' ears some variation on the theme, "You are perfect exactly the way you are, except do it better." Only now, I can add a little wine and a dance move and lovingly shout, "Life is short, y'all . . . take a sip!"

But, in all seriousness, you guys? Yoga is intimidating and challenging, especially your first time. No one ever said it wasn't. But it does get easier. All it takes is perseverance. Through repetition we find insight. And if you keep coming back to class, repeating those poses and refining those transitions, one day, many weeks, months, or perhaps even years later, you'll finish a class without breaking a sweat and think, "Huh. That was . . . pretty smooth. *And* enjoyable."

Just like sex. Wait, I mean . . . Ugh, fudge. Sorry. Did I just ruin the metaphor? JK #*nailedit*

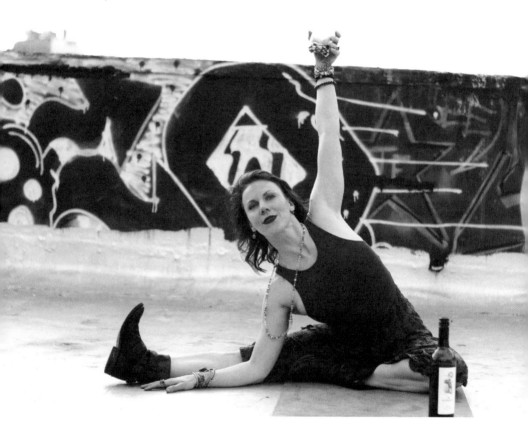

SOBER YOGA: SIDE-ANGLE POSE
SANSKRIT: *Parsvakonasana*

Drunk Yoga®: Pass-the-Chianti-Ya?

Emphasis on the upward inflection of the word *ya* should sound Canadian, or native of Northern Wisconsin,* where wine consumption is a right, not a privilege.

From downward-facing dog, bring your right foot forward and place it next to the inside of your right hand. Spin your left heel down so that your entire left foot is situated at a 90-degree angle, with your toes and front hips facing the left-side wall. Your arms are straight and parallel to the ground. Your shoulders are relaxed and stacked over your hips, while your gaze is forward, just beyond your wine. Once again, your right knee is directly above your right ankle, forming a stable 90-degree angle at the joint.

Place your glass of wine on the outside of your right foot. Place your right hand inside your right foot or, if that isn't accessible, simply place your right forearm on the top of your right thigh. Bring your left arm up and over your head, so that your left fingertips reach toward the ceiling and your gaze follows.

After an optional vinoyasa, repeat on the left side.

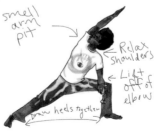

---

*I can say this because I'm from Wisconsin.

*Drunk Yoga®: Drunk Lunge**

From downward-facing dog, bring your right foot forward, inside your right fingertips.

Keep your back heel lifted and reaching back as you engage the muscles of your leg.

Make sure your right knee is directly over your ankle and you're curling your hips slightly forward to avoid sinking or hyperextending.

Your spine is long and straight. Keep your arms aligned with your ears as your fingertips reach toward the sky.

If you're bending your elbows like a cactus, take a moment to pause and ask yourself, "Am I a cactus?" And if the answer is "No," then check yo'self.

If the answer is "Yes," then, please, continue.

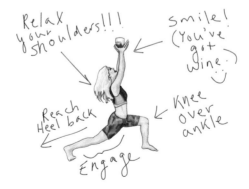

---

* *As opposed to "high" lunge. (#getit?)*

Drunk Yoga®: Ardha Hanuma-hiccup-asana

From croissant lunge, lean back onto your back shin. Flex your front foot as you extend your front leg and engage your muscles.

Lean forward but lead with your heart to avoid rounding your upper back.

Relax your shoulders.

Crawl your fingertips in front of you and press the top of your back foot into the ground to avoid putting too much pressure on your back knee.

Breathe.

Know that this pose was named after a monkey god and allow that visual to make you chuckle.

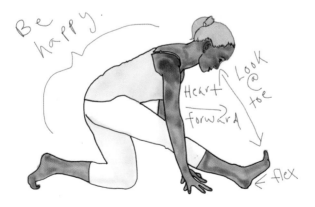

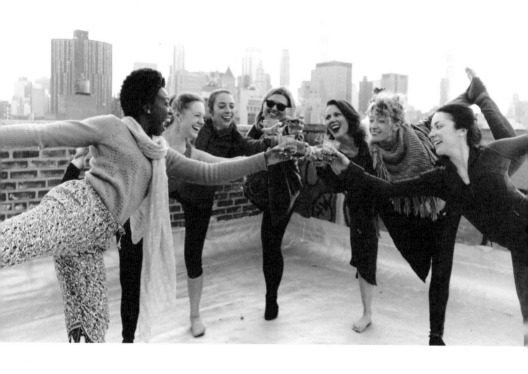

DRUNK YOGA® ETIQUETTE

1. Remove shoes. (Socks okay, but not if they smell terrible.)

2. Keep cell phone on and take as many photos as you can and tag @drunkyoga, k thanks.

3. Arrive exactly on time so you don't miss happy hour.

4. Don't skip sauv-asana. (Everybody loves a good wine-nap.)

5. Respect the teacher's sequencing. Unless you feel you can't do a pose, don't want to do a pose, or have any better ideas, then you do you, man.

6. Don't try to impress anyone. (Believe me, no one is impressed.)*

7. Put your props away after class: clean up your wine spills, put your glass back on the bar, roll up your mat, and high-five the teacher on the way out!

8. "Mi bar floor es tu bar floor," yes, but respect the space. ("An attitude of gratitude is the highest yoga," says everyone who knows anything about nothing[ness].)

9. Honor your limits (both bodily and fluids).

10. Practice eye contact with at least two people per class, held for at least three seconds each (with consent; otherwise that would be weird).

11. Meet someone new.

12. No "wine-ing." (Nobody likes a wet blanket. Not even if it's from a wine spill.)

(Continued on next page)

13. No saying the word "*yassss*." (I'm just . . . over it.)

14. Pretend you're sipping a glass full of giggles and laugh as much as possible.

15. Dance. Especially when everybody is watching.

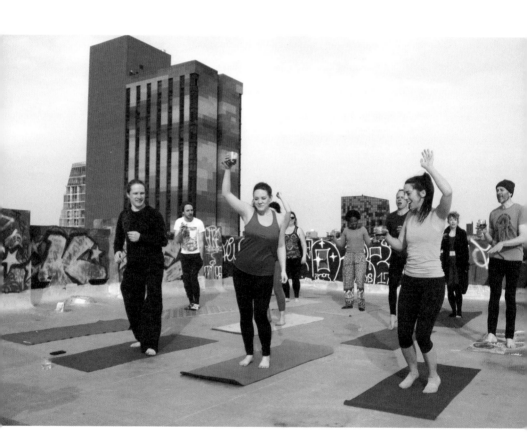

---

*JK you're so impressive omg.

HIGHLY SCIENCE-Y/ MATHEMATICAL FLOWCHART

I know very little about science, and math gives me brain freeze, but because yoga doesn't discriminate, I've created this easy-to-read flowchart about *balance*. You're welcome!

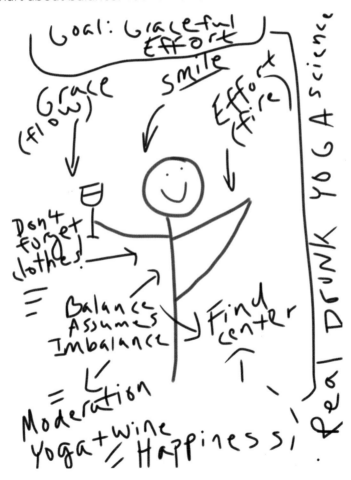

Drunk Yoga®: Chianti-konasana

Bring your right foot inside your right hand at the top of the mat. Spin your left heel down to a 90-degree angle. Straighten your right leg without hyperextending. Place your right hand on your right shin, on the ground inside your right shin, or a few inches off the ground inside your right shin with your outer right wrist pressing against your leg.

Raise your left arm to the sky and allow your gaze to follow. If you want to feel fancy, you can raise your glass of wine into the air by holding it in your left hand, but any effect it has on your experience of this pose as far as "fancy feelings" are concerned is strictly placebo.

Hey! You! Yes! You! Stop hunching your shoulders by your ears. I can see you doing it from over here.

Lengthen through the crown of your head and breathe.

Relax those shoulders, friends. We *just* went through this.

After about five breath cycles, release into *vinoyasa*. From downward-facing dog, move to the left side.

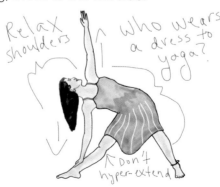

SOBER YOGA: CROW POSE
SANSKRIT: VAKASANA

Drunk Yoga®: Bakasana

Crow pose is a more advanced yoga pose and should be tackled with care.

Start in a squat. Bring your knees into your armpits and place your hands on the ground about eight inches in front of each foot. Spread your fingers wide, look forward, and start to slowly lift your hips up. Shift the weight into the balls of your feet, and then your hands. Continue to keep your gaze forward, and if you feel you have enough strength, you may work toward bringing one, and eventually both, feet off the ground to touch.

Easy-peasy for you? Holding crow pose like a champ? Well, then try taking a sip through your (reusable/biodegradable) straw while holding the pose, and then we'll really start to humble that ego.

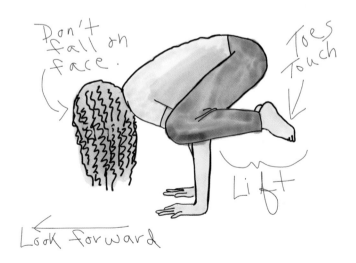

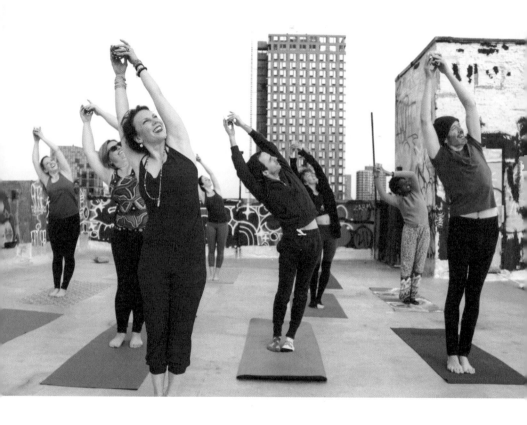

How to Get Up on the Downside of Yoga

Sober Yoga Pros

1. Detoxifying.
2. Stress-relieving.
3. Flexibility-enhancing.
4. Teaches self-reflection.
5. Strength-building.

Sober Yoga Cons

1. Competitive (be wary of the Instagram).
2. Addictive.
3. Expensive (you have to buy a *mat* and . . . actually, that's it, but still).
4. May lead to anxious, self-conscious thoughts about what others think.
5. May lead to spiritual obsession slash losing touch with reality.

Drunk Yoga® Pros

1. *Super* fun.
2. Stress-relieving.
3. Also detoxifying (in its own sort of "retoxifying" way).
4. Support of community.
5. Uninhibiting—> enhances self-esteem.

Drunk Yoga® Cons

1. You might have so much fun that you forget to be worried about that thing you were worried about.
2. You might spill wine on your shirt.
3. You might subsequently develop a love for a daily sober yoga practice and then have *one more thing* you've gotta fit into your busy schedule. *Ugh.*
4. You might laugh so hard that your face hurts the next day.
5. (I can't think of anything else.)

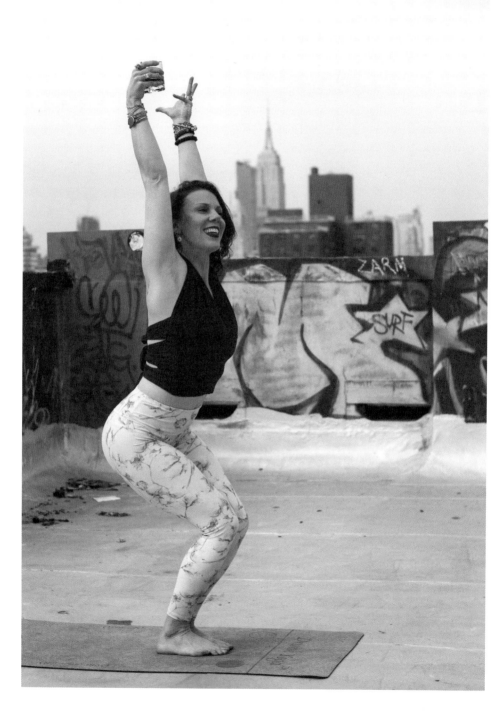

SOBER YOGA: CHAIR POSE
SANSKRIT: UTKATASANA

Drunk Yoga®: Ut-brut-asana

Nobody likes this (very dry) pose, so let's just get this over with.

Separate your feet hips-width distance, bend your knees, and stick your butt* out like you're about to sit on a miniature barstool behind you. Shift your weight into your heels.

Reach your arms up.

Relax your shoulders!

Rotate your armpits in toward your heart.

Relax your shoulders!

Lift your heart toward the sky to counter the urge to hunch your upper back and . . .

. . . oh for the love and God and all that is holy, relax your gosh** darn shoulders!

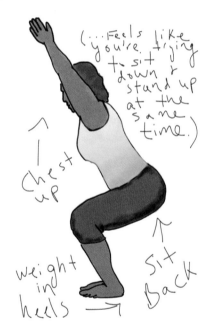

(...Feels like you're trying to sit down & stand up at the same time.)

↑
Chest up

↑ Sit Back

weight in heels →

---

* @$$
** godd@mn

Drunk Yoga®: Grenache-asana

From chair pose (page 55), cross your right leg over your left, and your right elbow underneath. If possible, wrap your right foot around your left calf and your right hand around your left wrist to really seal the deal.

Once you have accomplished a sense of stability in squeezing your centerline, while lifting off of each point of contact, sit a little deeper, raise your heart a little higher, and then yes, okay, fine . . . take a sip. #treatyoself

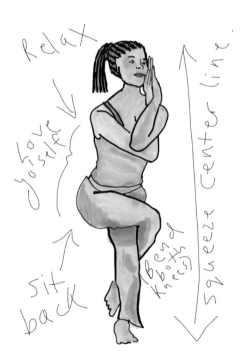

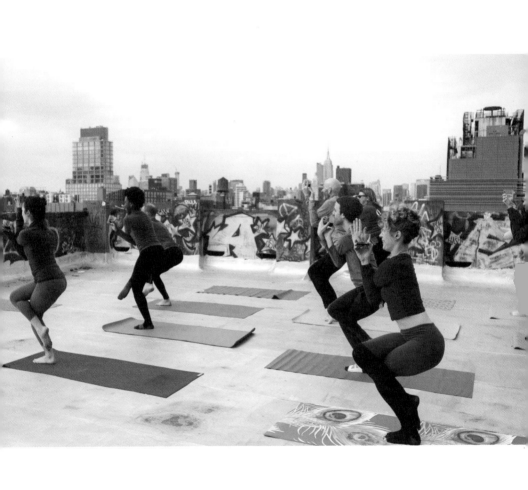

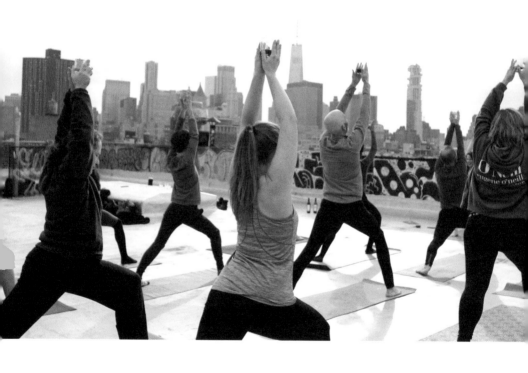

Top 10 Excuses
Not to Do Yoga

1. I'm not flexible. (Um . . . that's why you do yoga.)

2. I'm too busy. (Too busy for long-lasting health and happiness? *False.*)

3. I'm too old.

4. It's not my thing. (You make a good point.)

5. My goldfish wanted me to sleep in. (Goldfish can be persuasive, so I'll give you that one.)

6. Yoga is for girls. (What is this, 1927? Oh wait, women weren't allowed to do yoga until 1937. Until then, ashrams were "Broga" central. Nice try, though!)

7. I'm too tired. (Cough, Restorative Yoga, cough cough.)

8. I don't feel like it. (Buddy, nobody ever went to a yoga class and afterward said, "Man, I wish I hadn't done that." Just saying.)

9. I'm afraid I'll look stupid. (Honestly? You might. But that's what Drunk Yoga® is for. We'll all look stupid together. And, with our trusted vino-support system, we'll *think* we look *awesome.*)

10. 10a. Ugh, okay fine I'll go. (Listen, if you want to lead an enriched life, you need to learn how to develop techniques to cultivate personal joy. A ritualistic practice of gratitude and mindful movement allows you to appreciate . . .)

11. 10b. *I said I'll go.* (Oh! Great! Well then, namaste.)

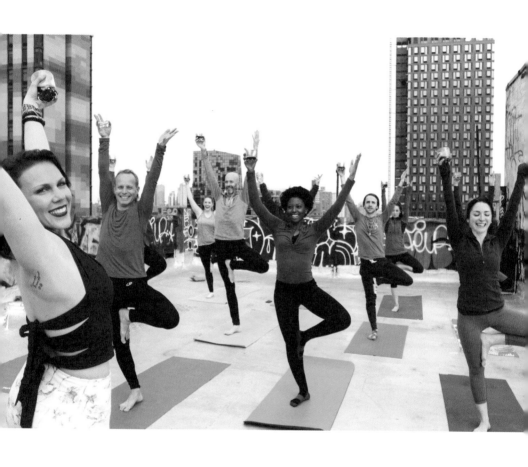

Drunk Yoga®: Chiant-tree Pose*

With your glass of wine in your left hand, use your right hand to grasp your right ankle and guide your foot up to your inner left thigh (alt. option: inner left calf). Bring both arms up and above the head and switch the glass of wine into the right hand, lowering both arms to parallel. Repeat three times. On the third time, bring the wine to heart center, and take a sip.

Yogi life hack: Press inner left thigh to right heel to find centerline and press through the left heel into the ground below you as you rise through the top of the head.

Once finished, cheers your neighbor, and move to the other leg. (A transitional sip is *optional* . . . but recommended . . .)

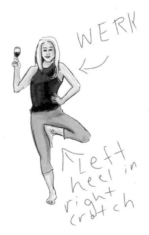

WERK

Left heel in right crotch

---

* For best results, drink Chianti. Or, actually, water. It's probably time that you hydrated. #detoxtoretox

Chiant-tree Buddy System

Find a partner. Do tree pose. Link arms. Take a sip. Boom. Done.

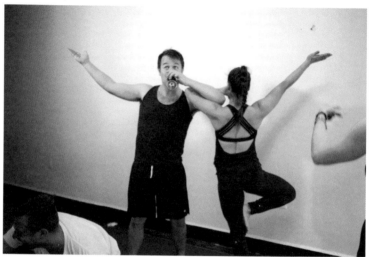

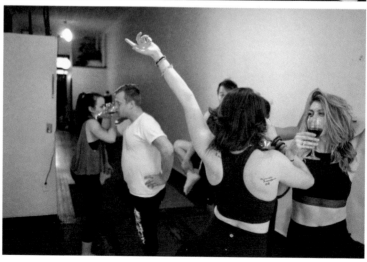

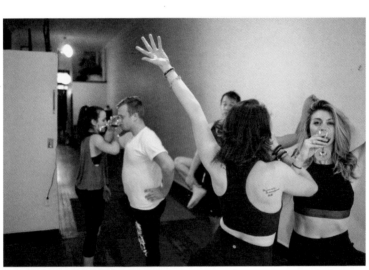

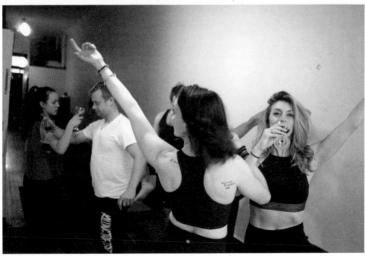

LIFT YOUR SPIRIT(S):
How to Set a Drunk Yoga® Intention

Setting an intention is my favorite part of yoga—"drunk" or "sober." Actually, it's my favorite part of waking up in the morning. And going to bed at night. And sitting for meditation. And taking a bath. And going on a trip. And buying a new dress. And making my bed (that one time I made my bed three years ago). And eating a vegan, gluten-free "cheeseburger," whether or not it's organic! (#jk #eatorganic #fosho) Anything and everything that has a beginning, middle, and an end is the perfect opportunity to set an intention.

FAQ

What's an intention?
It's direction with a purpose.

Why should I set an intention for a yoga class? Or bed making? Or shoe shopping?

Because anything done with intention gives it meaning—a reason for being. Without purposeful direction, your actions are aimless and your energy will be wasted. Like riding a bike for hours without knowing where you are going. Or driving a car when you're lost without stopping to type your destination into the GPS. First, you'll kill your hamstrings, and second, you'll burn through your gas. And for what?

Reminder

The only difference between a habit and a ritual is that a habit is done unconsciously, while a ritual is done with presence and purpose.

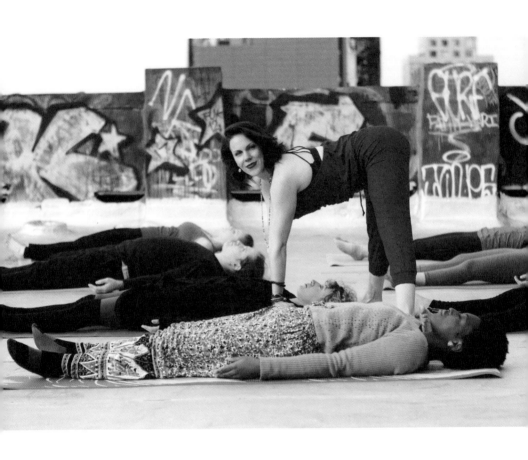

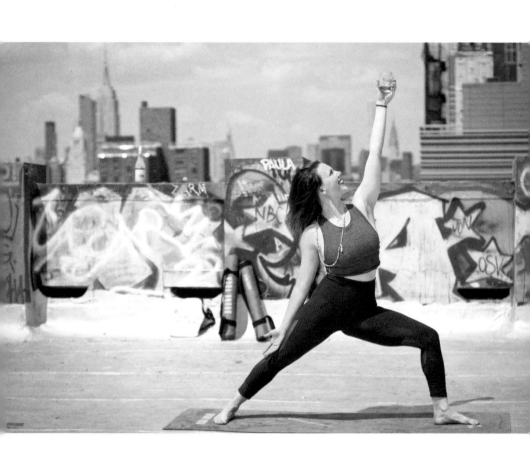

TIPSY TIPS FOR SETTING TERRIFIC INTENTIONS

- Know why you're doing what you're doing.

- Begin each activity with a pause, a breath, and conscious self-inquiry. Ask, "Why am I here on this yoga mat, in this class, with these people, at this time? What do I want to get out of this experience? How do I want to feel at the end? What do I need to let go of in order to achieve that goal?" With a glass of wine in your hand, you can imagine that you are magically setting this intention into the wine itself, so that as you sip throughout the class, you are sipping your way closer and closer to your goal. And of course, you can ritualize anything using the same model of self-inquiry, e.g., "Why am I adding marshmallows to my eggs for breakfast? How do I want to feel after this meal, and what do I need to let go of in order to achieve that feeling?" (Ahem . . . the marshmallows. Maybe let go of the marshmallows.)

- Know the end goal. You know, like, the meaning of life. #nbd

- For me, my larger purpose is joy. I make sure that every project I start is a path to joy. For every material object I purchase, I ask myself, "Will this bring more joy into my life?" And if the answer is "Yes," then I *will* buy that third Captain Planet coffee mug, thank you very much. And if I'm going to teach a class called "Drunk Yoga®," I will first make sure that my primary intention is to bring joy to others. But, that's just me. You may find that your heart's compass points toward peace, love, family, money, or even caring for your pet rocks. And that's fine! No judgment from the #drunkyogagirl. Just know why you're doing what you're doing, and what you want out of it, so you can live the richest, most consciously productive life you possibly can.

State the intention.

- Language is action. If the yoga teacher asks you to set your intention, allow the words to bubble up from your heart like a glass of very expensive champagne (because we don't want to set cheap intentions) and state your direction in your mind. "I'm letting go of fear." "I am happy." "I am free of stress." "I am the proud owner of three Captain Planet coffee mugs." (Just, you know, for example.)

You can change your mind.

- I understand that intention setting at the beginning of a yoga class can be a lot of pressure, mostly because the teacher only gives you like thirty seconds to do it. (Ugh, yoga teachers, amirite?) To take some of the pressure off, I'm here to tell you that although it is powerful to follow through on your goals, you can give yourself permission to change your mind. For instance, say you come into a yoga class superstressed because your boss just sent you an email saying, "Come in to my office as soon as you get to work. We need to talk." And so your intention for the class may be, "Manifest a new job, ASAP." But, halfway through class, you remember that it's your coworker's birthday next week and that your boss just wants to talk to you about throwing her a surprise party. So, you can quickly change your intention to "Be present," or something superyogic like that.

Track your intentions.

- It can be helpful to set intentions on a schedule. I set a new intention for each week every Saturday evening, and I ritualize it by having a glass of wine (gasp!), listening to music, lighting a candle, and writing about my upcoming week's goals in my journal. Then, I write a specific, clear intention on a piece of paper and display it on my personal altar, adorned with stones, oils, sage, and little meaningful treasures from my travels.

- If you don't have an altar (because you're, you know, a normal human being with a rich social life), you can magnetize it to your fridge, or set it by your bed. For the following seven days, my intention remains more or less the same. So, if my week's intention is in the realm of radical self-care, in a yoga class my intention might be "give thanks to my body," cough hippie cough cough. And if in the same week I (consciously) choose to binge-watch the newest season of *Orange Is the New Black*, my intention might be "rest and rejuvenate."

- I also have friends who work with the cycles of the moon. (And by "friends," I mean "me.") On every new moon, I reflect on my progress of last month's goals, and on every full moon, I set broader intentions for the upcoming month.

The reason for intention setting is to give yourself an opportunity to have the best experience possible with the task at hand. Be honest with yourself about your needs and be kind in tending to them. And if you can't think of an intention, you can always ask yourself, "What would Captain Planet do?" (No? Just me?)

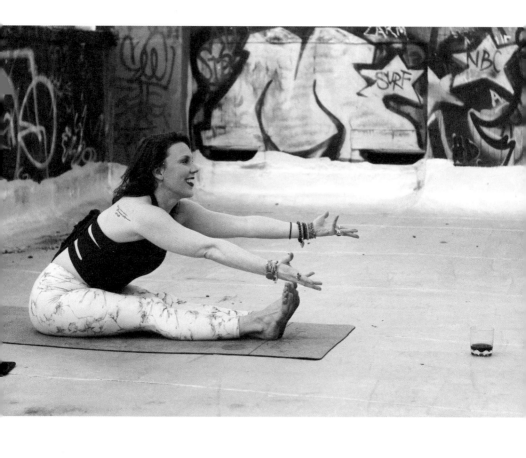

Happiness Checklist

(Things you can do besides Drunk Yoga®
—or sober yoga, for that matter—to build a joyful life)

1. Learn to sew so that you can make the DIY full-body sloth costume for Halloween you've always wanted.

2. Ring your neighbor's doorbell, and when they open the door, bop them lightly on the head and scream, *"Tag you're it,"* and then slowly, quietly, walk away, while maintaining eye contact. (Fun for the whole family!)*

3. Eat dessert before dinner. And then also *for* dinner.

4. Try something new! Like trapeze, white-water rafting, or calling your Uncle Herman from South Carolina and *not* engaging in a conversation about politics. #takeasip

5. Accidentally on purpose leave your cell phone at home while you roller-skate to the nearest hillside to watch the sunset. (You can take off the roller skates when you get to the hillside. Or don't. . . . If struggling makes you happy.)

6. Cuddle with a loved one. Pets are allowed . . . as well as pillows and childhood stuffed animals.

7. Take a bubble bath in the middle of the day while listening to the "Banana Boat" song.

8. High-five the traffic cop.

---

* Optional: Do this while wearing sloth costume.

9. Adopt a turtle and have a conversation with it in a made-up language of your choice.

10. Say the word "bubble" while sternly furrowing your eyebrows and try not to laugh.

11. _____

12. _____

13. _____ <— Now you try!

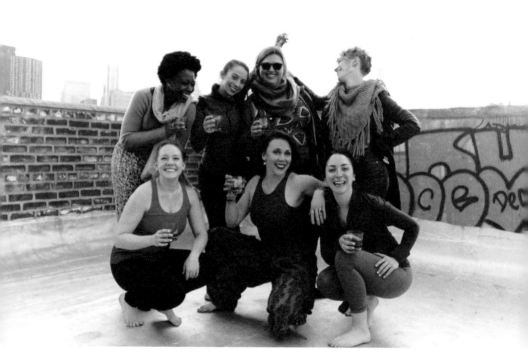

SOBER YOGA: LIZARD POSE
SANSKRIT: *UTTHAN PRISTHASANA*

Drunk Yoga®: Utthan Pri-Syrah-sana

Bring your right foot forward to the outer edge of the right side of the mat, next to your outer right hand.

Bend your right knee so that it is aligned directly on top of your ankle.

Ideally, keep your left leg extended backward with your heel and knee lifted. Another option is to bring your back knee down to the mat.

Bring your forearms down to the mat, with your elbows in line with the heel of your right foot.

Feel your collarbones reaching out to either side, so you keep your heart and gaze moving forward, rather than down into the abyss of your crotch.*

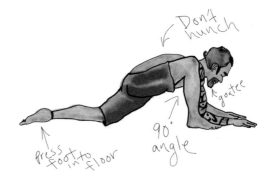

Don't hunch

goatee

90° angle

press foot into floor

Breathe here. Know that you chose to do Drunk Yoga® today, and so this discomfort is nobody's fault but your own.

When you're ready, vinoyasa/downward-facing dog, and try this on the left side.

---

* No new information there.

SOBER YOGA: WIDE-ANGLE SEATED FORWARD BEND
SANSKRIT: *UPAVISTHA KONASANA*

Drunk Yoga®: Ugh-ah-yeesh-ah-ko-nah-son-of-a . . .

There are two ways to do this pose: the fun way, and the "only-fun-for-contortionists" way.

I'll let you decide which is which.

Option #1

Open your legs wide and flex your feet. Lean forward with your heart and lead with the front of your pubis. Crawl forward with your hands. You can do that thing where you put your wine a few feet in front of you and try to reach for it (if your glass isn't already empty, that is).

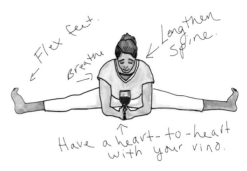

Flex feet.

Breathe

Lengthen spine.

Have a heart-to-heart with your vino.

Option #2

Same thing, but now you're balancing on your sitting bones while grabbing your big toe with the yogi toelock on each hand. It is important here that as you balance (and by balance, I mean wobble), you lift through your chest to avoid compressing your vertebrae. Engage

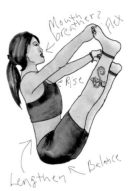

Mouth breather?

Flex

Rise

Lengthen

Balance

your abdominal muscles and use your arm strength to draw your legs in closer. Fall over, if you must, but be sure to laugh at yourself if you do. (Because, come on . . . it's just yoga.)

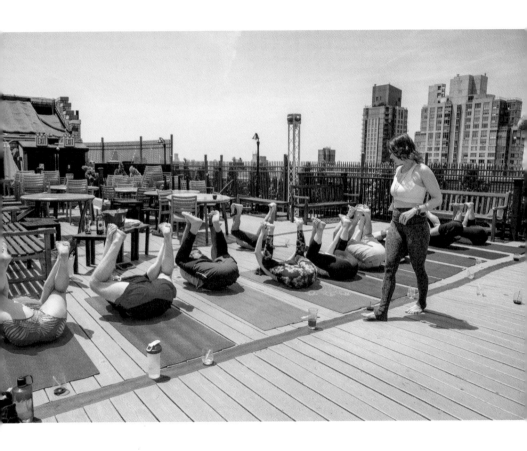

Drunk Yoga®: Same as Sober Yoga

A standing, wide-legged pose that will challenge your muscles, your mind, and your PC muscles.

Separate your feet wide on the mat and turn them out like a ballerina.

Bend your knees. Engage all of the . . . well, everything.

Bring your hands to your heart center and make effort to straighten your back/spine.

Want to take it up a notch? Extend your arms out to your sides, parallel to the ground, as if you are trying to push the walls away from you. If it helps, pretend you're Wonder Woman and that it's actually working. (Warning: it won't work.) Do you want to know what *does* work? Pelvic thrusting like you're in a 1980s workout video with Jamie Lee Curtis. No, really. Just try it.

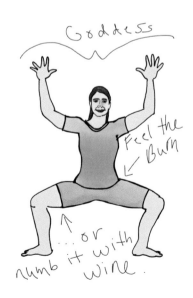

Release after several cycles of breath.

Pop a (Goddess) squat and take a sip. You've earned it!

#NAMASTERESPONSIBLY

(A message on healthy boundaries and moderation)

The healthiest life is one conducted in moderation. Even moderation is healthiest in moderation.

Yoga makes you feel fantastic. But like anything *fantastic*, the yoga "high" we often begin to crave after really digging in to a yoga routine can be addicting. And then we practice too much yoga. And then we get tired. And then we start to resent yoga. And, you guys, yoga didn't do anything to deserve that, now did it?

Another huge risk of getting addicted to yoga is developing what I like to call a "spiritual ego." Cue next slide. (Ahem, see next page.)

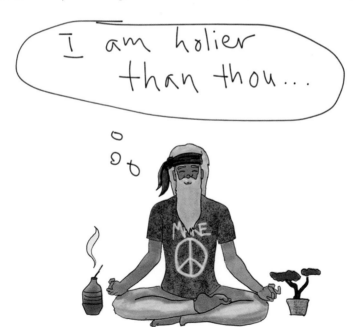

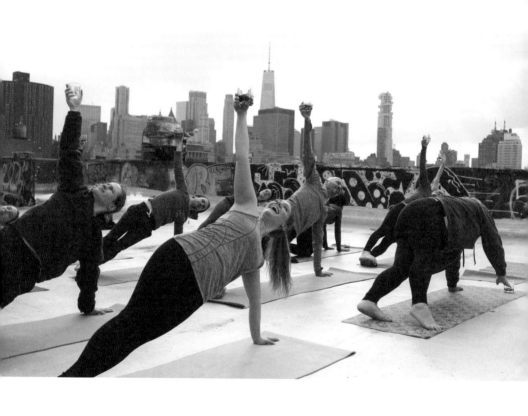

SOBER YOGA: SIDE PLANK
SANSKRIT: VASISTHASANA

Drunk Yoga®: Vino-sassy-nah*

From plank pose, shift your weight onto your right hand and position your body so that it is perpendicular to the ground, with the outer edge of your right foot pressing into the mat.

As you lift your left arm into the sky, don't forget to bring your wine with you, because, um, hi . . . this is Drunk Yoga®.

Engage your core, and draw your pubis, navel, and sternum forward to create a hint of a backbend.

Shift your weight ever so slightly into the first-finger knuckle of your right hand and feel like you're lifting off of the contact that your hand is making with the ground. In other words: lift—don't sink.

Hold for thirty minutes.

Just kidding.

No, but seriously.

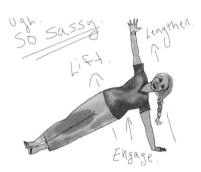

After thirty minutes (give or take twenty-nine minutes), gently place the glass down as you return to plank pose to repeat on the left side.

---

* This pose is for intermediate to advanced yogis. Sassiness and/or vulgarity is excused for beginners and women over the age of fifty in this pose.

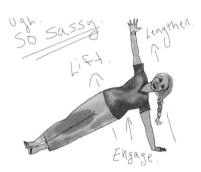

FIVE-POINTED STAR

Its open stance feels expansive, and it is often considered to be a pose that brings joy.

I teach this to elementary school children, which actually has a lot of crossover to Drunk Yoga®, as far as behavioral tendencies and fart jokes are concerned.

Stand on your mat, spread your legs and arms out wide, and lengthen in every direction at once.

On the count of three, shout the name of something in your life you'd like to let go of.

If you can't think of anything in your life you'd like to let go of because, oh, I don't know, you're just an extraterrestrial visiting us from another planet where nothing bad ever happens, then you can simply shout the name of a food that you'd most like to eat in this moment.

. . . 1

. . . 2

. . . 3

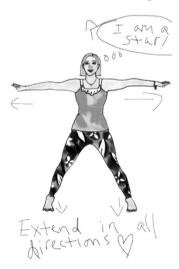

Vegan, gluten-free mac and cheese! (I'm not an alien . . . just a hippie with low blood sugar and the drunchies.)

Drunk Yoga®: Not-a-Rioja-jasana*

This pose is a toughie. Let's start with the right leg.

Balancing on your right leg in a standing position, bend your left knee and grab the inside of your left foot with your left hand.

Slowly start to lean forward.

As you reach forward with your right hand/glass of wine, kick into your left hand with your left foot.

Balance. You are a beautiful dancer. High five. Or, cheers, rather.

Release. Shake out your right leg. Do a little dance, perhaps, and then move onto your left side.

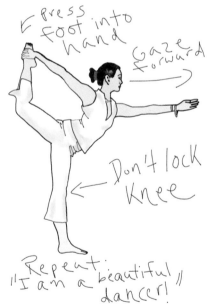

Press foot into hand

Gaze forward

Don't lock knee

Repeat: "I am a beautiful dancer!"

---

* Just . . . so we're clear.

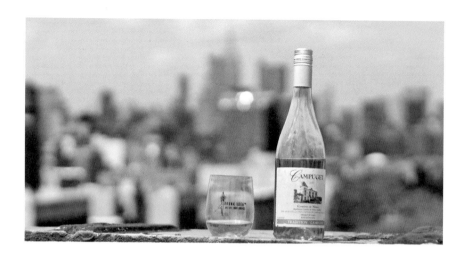

MAKE LIKE A ROSÉ AND CHILL

(Nine reasons not to take ~~yoga~~ life too seriously)

1. Nobody gets out alive.

2. Life doesn't take *you* seriously, so . . .

3. Because that's what they *want* you to think.

4. Life is just a temporary condition. This too shall pass. And by "this" I mean you, and everything and everyone you hold dear. Space dust. We'll all turn into space dust and *die*.

5. We're all one in love, guys, amirite?

6. If you can't stand on your hands, you're still a good person (probably).

7. Not to harp on the farting in yoga thing, but everybody does it.

8. We all put our pants on one leg at a time (especially super-tight yoga leggings).* Who cares if you can't touch your toes?

9. I am nobody. Nobody is perfect. Therefore, I must be perfect.

Here are some quotes on the matter from some pretty average people you've probably never heard of:

"Failure is the condiment that gives success its flavor."
—Truman Capote

"Don't go around saying the world owes you a living. The world owes you nothing. It was here first."
—Mark Twain

"Man suffers only because he takes seriously
what the Gods made for fun."
—Alan Watts

"Train yourself to let go of everything you fear to lose."
—Yoda

"Frame your mind to mirth and merriment
which bars a thousand harms and lengthens life."
—William Shakespeare

"Nonsense wakes up the brain cells. And it helps develop a sense of humor, which is awfully important in this day and age. Humor has a tremendous place in this sordid world. It's more than just a matter of laughing. If you can see things out of whack, then you can see how things can be in whack." —Dr. Seuss (<— I am pretty sure he was referring specifically to Drunk Yoga® when he came up with this one.)

---

* Except if you're good at yoga. Then you can put your pants on *both* legs at a time. With eyes closed. On the count of three breaths. #goals.

Drunk Yoga®: Urdhva Prosecco and something-something-asana*

With your right foot at the top of the mat, launch off your back foot to raise your left leg toward the ceiling, balancing your weight on your right leg.

Keep your right leg muscles very engaged, and microbend your right knee.

If you're feeling frisky (and you *are*), you may consider bringing one hand, or even both hands, behind your right calf/ankle.

Keep your gaze looking down.

Point your left toes.

Great. Now, all that's left to do is enjoy!

. . . And when you're no longer enjoying it, float your left leg down. Take a moment to forward fold, and then repeat on your left leg.

Oh, you're still enjoying it? Then by all means, continue. I'll wait.

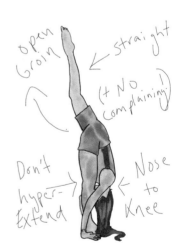

open Groin

← straight

(+ NO. complaining!)

Don't hyper-→ Extend

Nose to Knee

---

* Essentially, the splits, but while balancing on one leg. #nobigdeal

Drunk Yoga®: "Argh! Ah! Shandra!"-sana*

Place your right hand about 10 inches in front of your right foot. Launch off your left foot and shift all of your weight onto your right foot, bringing your left leg parallel to the ground. Your front-side body faces the left wall as your left arm rises.

If you forgot to take your wine with you on this one, don't worry about it. Just focus on *relaxing your shoulders* and flexing your left foot as you engage your back leg.

Don't lose your balance.

. . . And when you *do* lose your balance, release the pose.

Take a sip.

Try the left side.

. . . Or, don't. Whatever. If you're going to sit there and "wine" about it, see if I care.

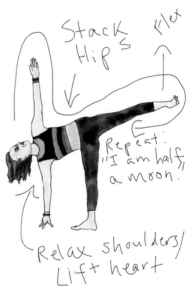

Stack Hips

Flex

Repeat: "I am half a moon."

Relax shoulders/ Lift heart

---

* Pretend you have a friend named Shandra and you're annoyed because they just finished off the bottle.

"One is more flexible when drunk."

Still today, a favorite journalist interview question for Drunk Yoga® is "Does wine help with flexibility?"

So, naturally, I Googled it.

And the answer(s) I found?

Nobody knows.

There is no shortage of online articles that discuss the topic of "wine health," but they all seem to come to contradictory conclusions based on various cited scientific studies.

So here's my thoughts on the matter (and you can alert the media!):

The *purpose* of yoga is not about gaining flexibility of the body, and neither is drinking wine—much less the experience of mashing them both together.

I have observed and experienced that lubricating oneself with vino during *vinyasa* can certainly make one feel more relaxed, which can, subsequently, make one feel more malleable. But if you do seek to increase your flexibility in a lasting way, you need to commit to stretching (and/or practicing yoga) regularly, not just once in a while in a bar with your friends at my superawesome happy fun class. (Did I mention that I teach Drunk Yoga®?)

Furthermore, the *purpose* of Drunk Yoga® is less about the physical benefits of yoga and wine—though there are many—and more about feeling great about yourself as you try something new surrounded by positive people.

Example (pulled from *Refinery29*):

"When the class ends, one of the other students, K. Bevin Ayers, thirty, an actress, tells me, 'It requires a certain amount of presence' to coordinate between sipping and yoga-ing. 'I wasn't going deeper into poses because of the alcohol, but I was connecting with my breath better.' She adds, 'I almost felt proud of how far I could go instead of being self-conscious.' (I, too, found myself more able to focus on the poses after a few sips.)"

In conclusion, in Drunk Yoga® as in life, it's all about balance, my friends. . . . in yoga *and* in wine.

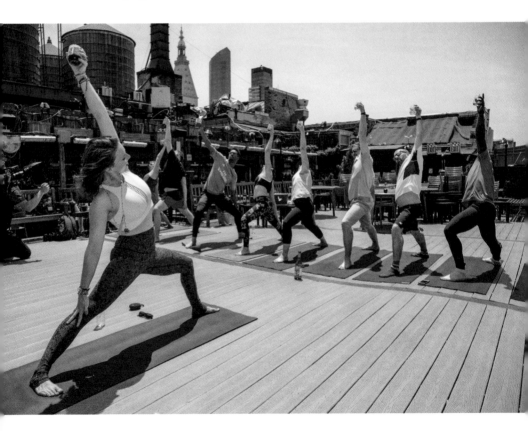

Drunk Yoga®: "Retox to Detox"

Bend your right knee and bring your right foot to the left edge of the mat, so that your knee is pointing toward twelve o'clock.

Bring your left leg over your right, placing your left foot outside your right thigh. Your left knee points directly up toward the ceiling.

Sit up tall with a straight spine, tilting slightly forward on your pubis.

Here, you are flushing your liver, which never in the history of yoga has ever been more important than it is in this moment, so pay attention.

Place your right hand on the ground behind your sacrum for support and bring your left elbow outside your right knee. Using this contact as leverage, press your elbow into your knee and twist, looking over your right shoulder.

When you're ready, gently countertwist by looking over your left shoulder and then switch legs to repeat on the other side.

Shimmy your chest and legs in transition. I mean *really* shimmy.

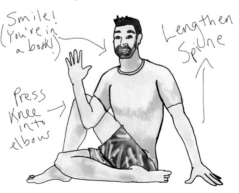

SOBER YOGA: CAMEL POSE
SANSKRIT: USTRASANA

Drunk Yoga®: Juice-drasana*

If you know you have lower-back issues, go ahead and sit this one out. Take a sip and enjoy while watching the rest of us struggle. I mean stretch.

Come to stand on your knees, hips-width apart.

Engage your butt** muscles and place your hands just above each butt*** cheek, framing your sacrum.

Guide your heart forward and up as you elongate your throat and look back.

All good? Okay, then you can slowly place your hands (one at a time) on your heels.

Continue to thrust**** your pelvis forward and your heart up.

Breathe.

When you're ready to release, gift yourself with a child's pose (page 8) and send some love to your lower back. Sippage of wine to follow.

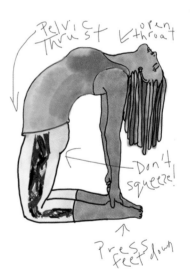

Pelvic Thrust
open throat
Don't squeeze!
Press feet down

---

* Because wine is essentially old grape juice, amirite?
** @$$
*** @$$
**** Let's do the Time Warp again.

WTF Are Chakras?

Let me 'splain. Chakras are known as the seven energy centers of the body, each correlating with various specific aspects of our physical, mental, emotional, and spiritual health. Here's my "beginner Drunk Yoga® guide" to chakras. Ahem:

Root Chakra

Sanskrit name: *Muladhara*, meaning root or support

Location: Between the anus and the genitals

Associated color: Red

Main issues: Survival/physical needs, such as security and shelter

Root chakra in balance: You did your laundry, you got a raise at work, you paid your rent, and now you're curled up on your couch eating (vegan, gluten-free) lasagna, binge-watching Netflix.

Root chakra out of balance: You've run out of underwear, you can't afford rent, you got kicked off your parents' health insurance, and all the food in your fridge is moldy. Actually, your fridge is moldy.*

---

* This is a.k.a. "being 26 years old."

Sacral Chakra

Sanskrit name: *Svadhisthana*, or "sweetness"

Location: Lower abdomen, between the navel and the genitals

Associated color: Orange

Main issues: Sexuality, emotional balance

Sacral chakra in balance: You feel emotionally stable because your romantic partner has showered you with gifts, including your favorite scented candles, a rose petal bath, and a box of chocolates. He/she has also surprised you with a trip to Cancún, and you are presently sitting on the beach watching the sunset (wine in hand) and you just had the best sex ever because he/she is more attentive to your needs than his/her own because he/she studies tantra. And during your postcoital cuddle, you start inexplicably sobbing, and he/she holds you in his/her arms and sweetly says, "It's okay. You can cry all you want. I'm here for you," which made you cry even harder. And then he/she handed you a tissue to blow your nose and wasn't weird about it at all.**

Sacral chakra out of balance: Examples include feelings of sex deprivation, PMS-ing, emotional eating, creative blockages, existential grief . . . yeah so . . . like, your average Thursday.

** Let me know if this person exists, yeah?

Solar Plexus Chakra

Sanskrit name: *Manipura,* or lustrous gem

Location: Between navel and base of sternum

Associated color: Yellow

Main issues: Personal power and self-will; self-esteem

Solar Plexus chakra in balance: You know what you want in life, you know why you want it, and you're not afraid to go out and get it because you got eight hours of sleep last night (fist bump) and you just had a double shot of espresso and you killed it in this morning's meeting and now you've decided to run for president (because wine not?) and actually now you're running a marathon, so yeah, okay, we'll talk later.

Solar Plexus chakra out of balance: I mean, everything is only temporary and then we die, so, like, what's the point? (*Goes back to bed. Gets out of bed, goes to kitchen, grabs ice cream from freezer, goes back to bed.*)

Heart Chakra

Sanskrit name: *Anahata,* or "unstruck"

Location: At the center of the chest

Associated color: Green

Main issues: Love and relationships

Heart chakra in balance: Examples include: 1. You just matched on Tinder with your college crush; 2. You're on your honeymoon and you think you're the luckiest, happiest couple in the world (give it a day, though, and we'll revisit the sacral chakra); 3. You just had a new baby and you're oozing love from every orifice; 4. Your puppy is cuddled up in your lap and you're choosing to be late for work because you don't want to disturb the little guy because this, *this* is love.

Heart chakra out of balance: All of the things that cause a human to be heartbroken. Examples include: 1. Your partner cheated on you; 2. You just got dumped; 3. Your sibling/parent/pet just died . . . sorry, is that depressing? Here, have some wine and get thee to thy yoga mat.

Throat Chakra

Sanskrit name: *Vishuddha*, or "purification"

Location: Centrally at the base of the neck

Associated color: Blue

Main issues: Communication and self-expression

Throat chakra in balance: As we yogis would say, "Speak your truth." And that is, of course, completely open to interpretation and is often used as a spiritual bypass in the yoga community. For example, you could say to someone you're dating, "Yes. I think your best friend is more conventionally attractive than you." And then quickly add, "But I'm just speaking my truth." To which they have no choice but to respond, "Um. Okay. Thanks for . . . being truthful." Now you try! Start with telling your boss what's *really* on your mind and let me know how it goes!

Throat chakra out of balance: Examples include: dishonesty, the inability to express how you really feel, a loss for words, verbal inhibition, or shyness. Conversely, you're extra gossipy and/or overly talkative with "no filter." See Youtube: "David After Dentist," for an example of a throat chakra that is perhaps a touch *too* open. (Though if there were ever an excuse to have no filter, dentist drugs would be it, 200 percent.)

Third Eye Chakra

Sanskrit name: *Ajna,* or to perceive, to know

Location: Above and between the eyebrows

Associated color: Indigo

Main issues: Intuition, wisdom

Third Eye in balance: A grounded connection to where mind meets matter. You're listening to your gut when it tells you, "Actually, I think I'm only going to law school because my parents want me to. I feel called to be an elementary school teacher." Or, "I feel like this relationship isn't a situation I am supposed to be experiencing right now. I think I need to travel and take some time to reflect." And, especially, "My intuition is telling me that I shouldn't get in that van with the man in a trench coat, even though I really want that candy he says he's got."

Third Eye out of balance: You're indecisive and aren't quite able to "go with the flow." You put too much weight on others' opinions of you, and you lack a sense of "purpose."***

*** Often a result of lack of sleep, overworking, or, dare I say it, too much wine. (You guys, moderation. We've been through this.)

Crown Chakra

Sanskrit name: *Sahasrara*, or "Thousand-fold"

Location: Top or crown of the head

Associated color: Violet, gold, white

Main Issues: Spirituality, depression, confusion, dementia

Crown chakra in balance: Examples include connection to spirituality, and a sense that you are a part of something greater than yourself—an "unseen" universality that feeds your soul and allows you to be present with "what is."****

Crown chakra out of balance: Examples include feeling depressed and purposeless. This often results from too much attachment to "the ego" and the material world. Try getting rid of all of your belongings, quitting your job, throwing your phone in the river, and changing your name to "Sri-Guru-Raja-Sushi-Tacos-Namaste-Feather-Lotus-Flower" and see if that helps.

**** Inaccessible through cheap wine. Go for the good stuff.

SOBER YOGA: RECLINED HERO POSE
SANSKRIT: *SUPTA VIRASANA*
Drunk Yoga®: Sip-da-vino-sana

Knees together, feet wide apart. Wineglass to your side. Sit in between your heels. If comfortable, you may recline back onto your elbows or lie down on your back.

If you have tight thighs, sit on a yoga block. Knee pain? Feel free to skip pose entirely. Chill.

Take a sip. Maybe lie back and catch a wine nap.

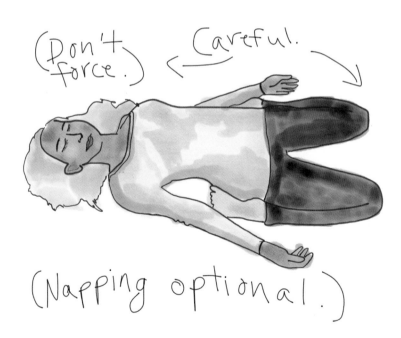

(Don't force.)   Careful.

(Napping optional.)

Drunk Yoga®: Cup-o'-tasana

Bring your right knee to the right edge of your mat at a 45-degree angle. With hips aligned with 3 o'clock and 9 o'clock, your left leg is long behind you and parallel to the edge of the mat.

Note that this is often a difficult pose. It can be painful, intense, and make you want to cry, swear, or groan. That's what the cup-o'-wine is for. #takeasip

And listen, if you need to support your right hip with a block, a pillow, or your cat, you may. Use what is available to you. (But make sure your cat gives you . . . ? That's right, friends. Consent.)

You may remain upright with your shoulders over your hips or crawl forward and rest your forehead on your hands.

Once you've found a comfortable, nay, tolerable position, find your breath. Give yourself a minute to be with your experience, without judgment or support of any particular thought or feeling.

And if you find that you have lulled yourself to sleep in this pose from the oceanic sound of your cyclical breathing, that's a good indication that you've taken a few too many sips and it's definitely time to call it.

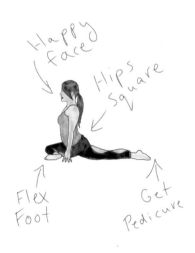

JOURNAL ENTRY PROMPTS

1. Assuming that nothing is divinely orchestrated and you are the maker of your own destiny and nothing happens for a reason and every mistake you've ever made to date is a result of your own mammalian-brained f*ckup, make a list of all of the things that give you an elusive sense of so-called purpose:

_____

_____

_____

_____

_____

_____

_____

_____

_____

_____

_____

_____

_____

_____

_____

_____

2. Now, assuming there is a higher power, and your individual fate *is* predetermined, and your existence has some great mysterious meaning, and everything that has ever happened in your life has occurred to bring you into perfect alignment, make a list of all of the things that bring you joy:

_____

_____

_____

_____

_____

_____

_____

_____

_____

_____

_____

_____

_____

_____

_____

_____

_____

_____

3. Your sense of personal identity is nothing more than an illusion. But *if* you *were* an "actual," "real" "person," what kind of an "impact" would you want your "existence" to have on the "world" and the other "people" in "it"?

4. Define "presence" and write about how it contributes to . . .

(Runs into the kitchen to pour a glass of pinot noir. Cuts finger on wine opener. Curses. Remembers why it's hazardous to drink and journal. Shrugs. Continues to pour.)

. . . a state of mental health and a sense of *(takes a sip)* overall well-being:

_____

_____

_____

_____

_____

_____

_____

_____

_____

_____

_____

_____

_____

_____

_____

5. If a tree falls in the forest, and no one is there to hear it, what is your favorite type of wine, and why?

_____

_____

_____

_____

_____

_____

_____

_____

_____

_____

_____

_____

_____

_____

_____

_____

_____

_____

_____

Drunk Yoga®: Go-moo-khasana*

Starting in a seated position, place your wineglass 1–2 feet in front of your mat. Tilt your pelvis forward and bring your right leg over your left so that your right knee is directly situated on top of your left knee. Both thighs are rotating inward. Shins are parallel to the top of the mat, and feet are flexed. Lead with your heart as you hinge from your hips and bend forward. Gaze is forward. Reach for your wine.

Eyes. On. The. Prize.

Lift chest

contemplate Pizza

Breathe

Squeeze inner thighs

Bonus Drunk Yoga®: The Corkscrew

Lean forward onto your fingertips. Stick your butt** in the air and, while on the balls of your feet, spin counterclockwise 360 degrees around yourself until you come back around in the same seated position ("go-moo-kasana") with your left leg on top.

Repeat the exercise.

---

* Dad joke.
** @$$

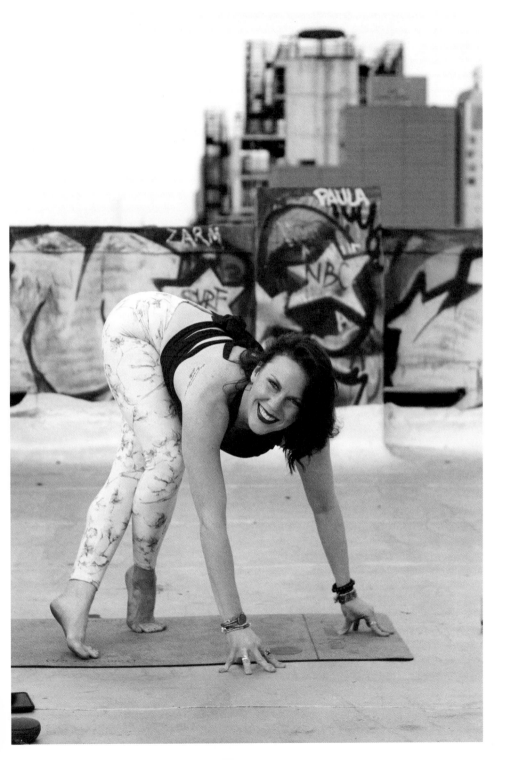

Drunk Yoga®: Nah-Syrah-sana*

From a seated position on your mat, lift your legs and torso to create a V-shape with your body.

Squeeze your legs together. If you want to look pretty, point your toes. If you don't, then . . . well, don't.

Arms are parallel to the ground, and your palms face each other.

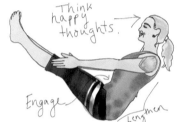

Engage your abdominal muscles by drawing your belly in toward your spine.

Lift through the crown of your head to lengthen your back and lift through your heart to avoid hunching the . . . For gosh** sakes. Relax. Your. *Shoulders*.

Bonus Drunk Yoga®: Boat Pose

With your glass of wine in your hand, separate your legs a few inches and figure-eight the glass in between your legs, switching the wine from one hand to the other. Laughing, singing, and grunting are not only allowed, but encouraged here. Just don't spill your wine. Because, I mean, what a waste.

---

* This pose is particularly for people who do not like Syrah.
**f#ck's

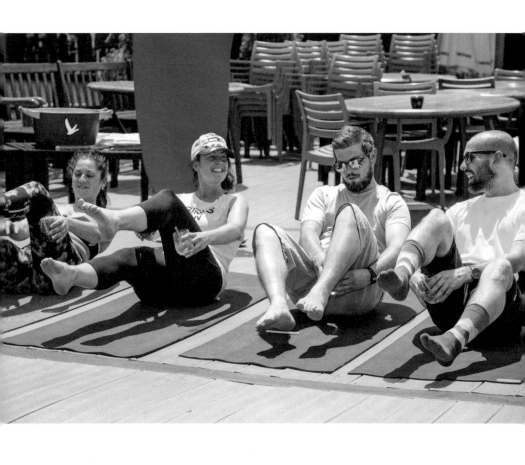

Drunk Yoga®: Pass-me-merlot-asana*

We're going to play that game again where we put the glass at least two feet in front of us and try to grab it, okay?

Extend your legs out in front of you, and then scooch** your butt*** back a couple of inches. This helps you ground onto your perineum rather than sit on your coccyx.

Leading with your heart, hinge forward from the hips and reach forward.

On the count of three, say the name of your favorite Spice Girl.

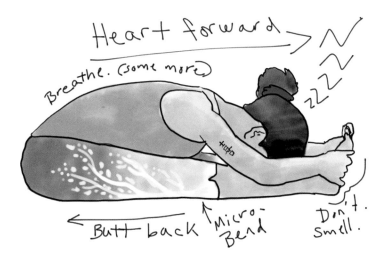

---

* For best results, use chardonnay
** Scientific term
*** @$$

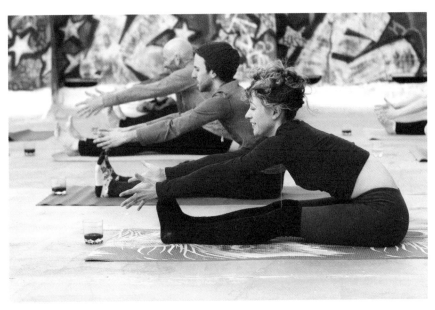

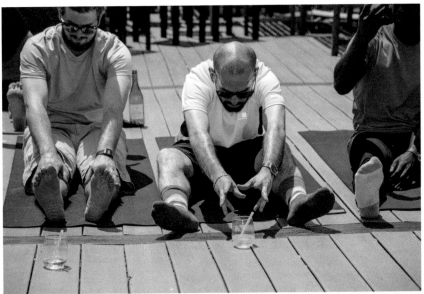

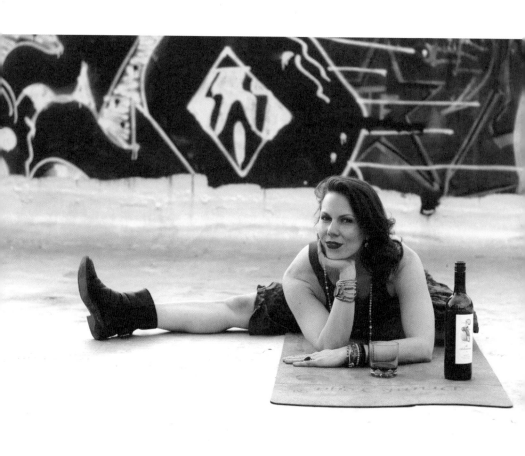

Sober Tips for a
Solo Yoga Practice

For those of you who already have a wonderfully dedicated home-practice, awesome! Great job! Good for you! You make up 1 percent of the population, and my best guess tells me you're a Virgo! But for the rest of us fiery-hearted, active-minded humans, it can be tough to keep a one-track mind on anything, much less *yourself* and your *breath* in conjunction with your *movement* on a *yoga mat* at *home* with your *laptop* and *TV* and *refrigerator* all just like, right there, rudely staring at you while you're trying to find enlightenment. *Ugh.* Here are some "Sober Tips" that might help you get started on your at-home yoga practice! (#MustNotLetRefrigeratorWin.)

1. Start small
Start with five to ten minutes a day. Do cat/cow poses (page 22 & 32), child's pose (page 8), and downward-facing dog. Frame this time for yourself as a contained space to "feel friggin' awesome."

2. Create a space that you want to practice in
I never feel like doing yoga when my space is a total mess. Conversely, when I clear my external space of old crap, I'm able to do the same for my internal landscape. . . . "As above so below, as without so within," ya feel me? So, pick up your sweaty laundry, wash your dishes, light some incense, and pump up some sweet jams for your own little personal yoga party.

3. Make it a reward, not a chore
Any personal ritual is a "coming home" to yourself, and this includes your at-home practice. As soon as it becomes a chore, rather than a gift, however, the ritual is doing you a disservice. That said,

smart people who probably know what they're talking about say that it takes 21 days to form a habit. So developing a new daily ritual may feel strenuous at first. Strenuous like "Mom I don't *wanna* do my homework it's only *Saturday*" strenuous. But trust me, it's worth it. Talk to me in 22 days.

4. Nobody has to know

Nobody has to know *why* you suddenly started showing up at the office all shiny and happy—suddenly so cool, calm, and collected—ready to conquer the day like you're a gosh darn champion. They just need to know that you *are*. The fact that you warrior-pose* upon waking while you brew your morning coffee can be our li'l secret, big guy.

5. Stick to a script

After you get the whole "I practice a little yoga every day because it makes me feel great" thing under your belt, I recommend moving into the next phase of an at-home practice, which is "I practice the same sequence every day because it helps me track my progress." The more you practice the same yoga sequence, the more opportunity you have to refine it. And subsequently, you'll learn something new about yourself in relationship to your body and the space it inhabits. And this is the secondary reason we do yoga, right? (The primary reason being to look good in a tank top, obviously.)

---

* I just turned a noun into a verb. #sorrynotsorry

Extra Yoga, Easy on the Drunk

When more yoga than wine is needed to be a functioning human person every darn* day, here's some practical applications of your practice for yogis and non-yogis alike!

- Missed your train? Pause. Take a deep breath, inhale. Exhale. It's okay. You'll catch the next one. And once you've micromeditated on the train platform for peace and patience, might I suggest watching the infamous Youtube video "Goats Screaming Like Humans" to lift your spirits while you pass the time?

- Ugh, wake up with a stiff back? Reach your arms way up high and then fold in half from the hips and touch the floor as you bend your knees. Hang here for a few with your face between your legs. Should fix the problem.

- Coworker/mom/ex say something passive-aggressively insulting (again)? *Pause.* Remember that anger does nothing except make you age faster, and you don't have time for crow's-feet, amirite? Feel your feet on the ground. Take a deep breath. And respond with grace.

- Ugh, did you watch Fox News again? Go for a walk around the block, mindfully taking in all of the sights and sounds, and remind yourself of three, no, *five* things you're grateful for.

- Mind won't stop a-chattering? Turn off the TV/music/phone, put down the book, and drink some tea (or, I don't know . . . a glass of wine, perhaps) and watch the sunset. (It never disappoints.)**

---

* d@mn

** Except when it's raining, snowing, too windy, or you remember when someone told you that the beautiful orange/pink colors are a result of air pollution. (Did I ruin your moment? Fudge. Sorry.)

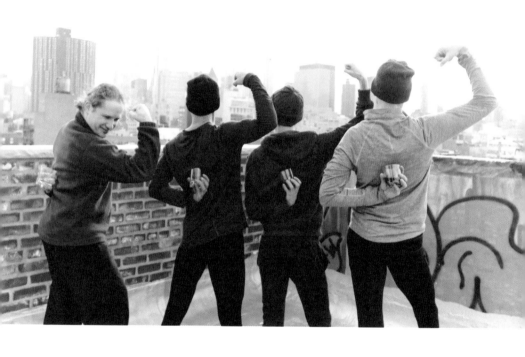

DRUNK BROGA

Drunk Yoga® is for your boyfriends.

You: "Baby, let's go to yoga together!"

Boyfriend: "No."

You: "Baby, let's go to yoga together!"

Boyfriend: "Not my thing."

You: "Baby, let's go to yoga together!"

Boyfriend: "No way. I can't even touch my toes."

You: "Baby, let's go to yoga together!"

Boyfriend: "I'd love to!" —> (and then you wake up from your dream and go to yoga alone . . . again)

You: "Baby, let's go to yoga together!"

Boyfriend: "We've been over this."

You: "There's wine."

Boyfriend: "Let's go."

Drunk Yoga®: Pour-the-Syrah-sana

From a seated position, place your palms by your hips, engage your core (*all* of it), and lift your hips. Gaze at the ceiling.

Take a big inhale . . .

And then exhale dramatically as you release back onto the ground.

(You did good, team. You did real good.) #takeasip

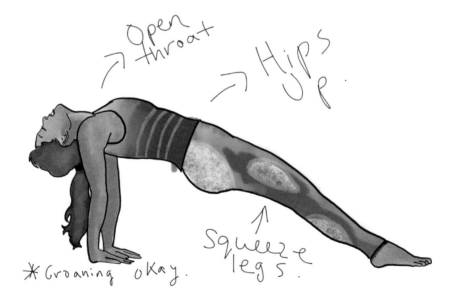

SOBER YOGA: BUTTERFLY POSE
SANSKRIT: BADHAKONASANA

Drunk Yoga®: Blanc-de-konasana

Place your wineglass a few inches in front of the top of your mat. Sit on the ground or the edge of a blanket with the soles of your feet together. Tilt your pelvis forward slightly for a better rotation of your hips. Actively press the soles of your feet together as you lean forward with your heart and vision, reaching for the wineglass.

If and only if you reach the wineglass, you may take a sip.

. . . Nobody likes a cheater.

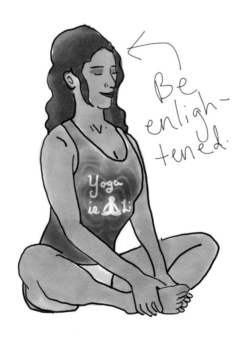

Be enligh-tened.

SOBER YOGA: SLEEPING TORTOISE POSE
SANSKRIT: *KURMASANA*

Drunk Yoga®: Kir-masana

Start in a seated position. Bring your legs out in front of you and slide your arms under each leg, until your shoulders are making contact with your knees.

Lean your heart forward to create a hint of a backbend.

You may rest your forehead on the ground, or place your glass of wine between your feet and take a sip once your face gets down there to reach it.

There's a bunch of ways to make the pose more difficult, but I won't do that to you, because I'm a nice person.*

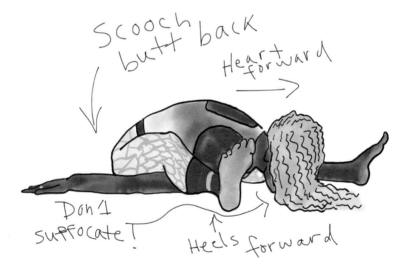

---

* . . . when I'm drinking wine.

SOBER YOGA: STAFF POSE
SANSKRIT: *DANDASANA*
Drunk Yoga®: Karaffe Pose

This one is fun for the whole family (whose members are 21+).

With your wine safely situated next to you on the mat, simply extend your legs long and place your palms down by your hips.

Gently press down through your palms, out through your flexed feet, and up through the crown of your head as you straighten your spine.

Breathe and enjoy this beginner pose while it lasts.

. . . Because it's all uphill from here.

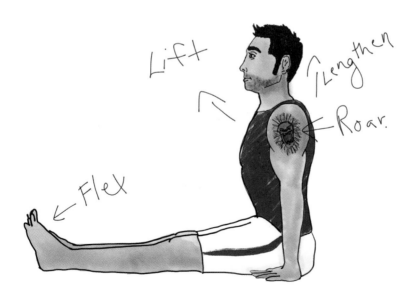

Drunk Yoga®: Juwanna-Syrah-sana

Extend your right leg out long in front of you on the mat. Situate your left heel in your right crotch (as opposed to the wrong crotch).

Hinging forward from your hips and leading with your heart, fold over your right thigh. If possible, wrap your hands around your right heel and touch your nose to your knee.

Involuntarily grunting from pain in body parts you didn't know you had? Don't worry. This pose, too, shall pass, and then we can all take a sip.

When you're ready, switch crotches and try this on the other leg.

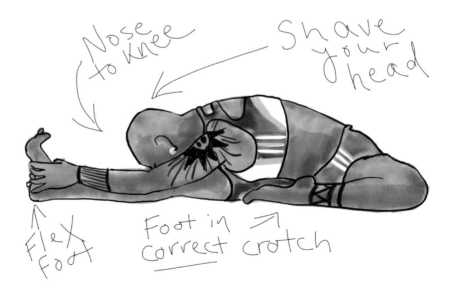

Drunk Yoga®: Brix Pose*

Begin lying on your back with your knees bent and feet flat on the ground, hips-width apart.

Press your feet into the ground as you lift your hips up. As you do this, scooch your shoulders close together and interlace your hands underneath you. Your throat should be slightly compressed here, with your chest pressing against your chin.

Engage your quads and abdominal muscles in this pose to maintain alignment.

Some yogis say you should *squeeze* your butt** muscles here to "protect your sacrum," and other yogis say you should *relax* your butt*** muscles here to "protect your sacrum." In conclusion: a lot of yogis have a lot of opinions. Try it both ways and have your own experience!

When you're ready to release from the pose, roll down from your shoulders slowly. Hug your knees into your chest to decompress your lower back and protect that beloved sacrum.

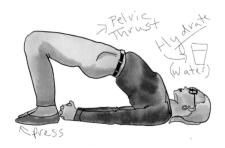

After you're finished here, don't take a sip. You've already had too many.

---

* Brix sounds sort of like "Bridge," and Brix is used to measure sugar in grapes that haven't been fermented yet. Don't believe me? Google it. ('Cause that's what I did!) #runningoutofwinepuns.
** @$$
*** @$$

AHEM. MORE YOGA. GLOSSARY

Noun: a word used to identify any of a class of people, places, or things

Verb: a word used to describe an action, state, or occurrence

Adjective: a word or phrase naming an attribute, added to or grammatically related to a noun to modify or describe it

Adverb: a word or phrase that modifies or qualifies an adjective, verb, or other adverb

Curse word: a solemn utterance intended to invoke a supernatural power to inflict harm or punishment on someone or something*

---

* Like @ss, and d@mn, sh!t, and all of those other words my editor doesn't want me to write.

AHEM. MORE YOGA.
FILL IN THE _____.

Once upon a time, there lived a middle-aged _____ (noun) _____ from __(noun) _____ named Mr. _____ (name) _____.

Mr. _____ had lower back pain from sitting at a computer all day long for years, a stiff ankle from an old track injury from high school, rug burn on both of his elbows from . . . well, it doesn't matter . . . not to mention a toothache. Looking in the bathroom mirror one morning, Mr. _____ spotted droopy _____ (noun) _____ under his eyes and permanent forehead wrinkles that seemed _____ (adj.) _____, which he was pretty sure weren't there the day before. (Can wrinkles appear overnight? Apparently so.)

Anyway, still looking in the mirror, Mr._____ declared to his reflection, "I'm not getting any younger. It's time for me to try yoga."

With conviction, he took a sip of _____ (noun) _____, gave the dog a _____ (adj.) _____ pat on the head, and exited the bathroom, ready to take on the day like a _____ (adj.) _____ champion. . . . Only to quickly realize he forgot to brush his _____ (noun) _____, so he _____ (verb) _____ back into the bathroom to finish the job.

After a long day at work, _____ (adverb) _____ typing _____ (noun) _____ while _____ (verb) _____ gently used bars of _____ (noun) _____ and ceramic tropical _____ (noun) _____, Mr. _____ threw on some sweat pants and a _____ (noun) _____, picked up a cheap yoga mat from the local _____ (noun) _____, and headed to the nearest yoga studio, which was cleverly named __(noun) _____.

Mr. _____ spent the first 10 minutes of class worrying whether he should take his socks off and whether his yoga mat was facing right-side up. But after the yoga teacher came over, knelt down beside

(Continued on next page)

him, and gently whispered in his ear, "Your yoga mat is upside down, and you should take your socks off," Mr. _____ gained clarity on both of those concerns, made the _____ (adj.) _____ corrections and climbed back into downward-facing _____ (noun) _____.

Looking around, Mr. _____ was _____ (adj.) _____, because everyone else in the class could get their heels on the ground and their bottoms up (cheers) at the same time, but he couldn't. His hands were _____ (adj.) _____, and his arms _____ (verb) _____. What the _____ (curse word) _____!?

However, he _____ (verb) _____. The class carried on, and Mr. _____ finally started to catch on to the whole "breathing in conjunction with movement" thing, and he felt pretty darn _____ (adj.) _____! And even though his _____ (noun) _____ were tired from all the _____ (adj.)___ poses, and he was self-conscious about having forgotten to wear _____ (noun) _____ because there was a very beautiful _____ (noun) _____ practicing next to him that he couldn't *not* notice, he realized his low back tension was starting to _____ (verb) _____ and his _____ (noun) _____ began to _____ (verb) _____. By the time he got to *savasana*, Mr. _____ was feeling _____ (adj.) _____ and _____ (adj.) _____. He didn't even _____ (verb) _____!

But, even though Mr. _____ left the studio that evening considering his first yoga class experience to have been an overall _____ (noun) _____, because he felt super Zen and _____ (adj.) _____, he still wasn't convinced yoga was "his _____ (noun) _____."

However, when we arrived home, and he saw that his dog had _____ (verb) _____ the _____ (noun) _____ in the _____ (noun) _____ like a __(adj.) _____ (noun) _____, he released a huge sigh and said, "_____ (curse word) _____, I need to go back to yoga."

SOBER YOGA: LEGS-UP-THE-WALL POSE
SANSKRIT: *VIPARITA KARANI*

Drunk Yoga®: See Sober Yoga

(. . . sounds pretty "drunk" to me)

Are you new to yoga? Did you mostly come here for the wine? Then this pose is for you.

Scooch your butt* up to the wall and extend your legs.

Lay with your arms out to your sides.

Close your eyes, focus on your breathing, or visualize something beautiful manifesting in your life, like a new romantic partner, a vacation to the tropics, or your loud neighbor who inexplicably moans to electronic music in the wee hours of the morning moving out so you can finally sleep in.**

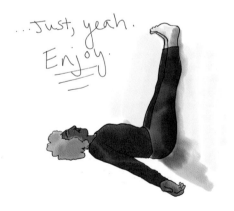

...Just, yeah. Enjoy.

---

* @$$
** No? Just me? Okay fine, then chocolate mousse cake. Visualize chocolate mousse cake.

SOBER YOGA: CORPSE POSE
SANSKRIT: *SAVASANA*

*Drunk Yoga®: Sauv-asana**

Lie flat on your back, palms faceup, legs splayed out, close your eyes, and allow yourself to surrender to gravity. Completely relax, letting go of your investment in being, doing, and having.

. . . And if your teacher is any good, they'll play a song like "Don't Worry, Be Happy" to help you feel *extra extra* at peace with your life . . . before you know it, you have to go back out in the world and deal with its inherent misery and inevitable suffering. (Ugh, sorry. Yeah, fine. Go ahead, take a sip.)

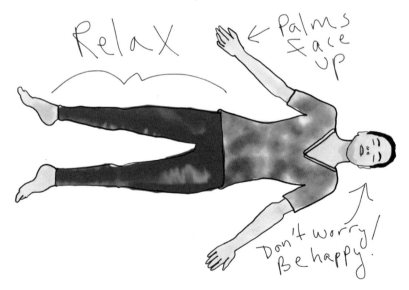

---

* Alt name: Wine Nap

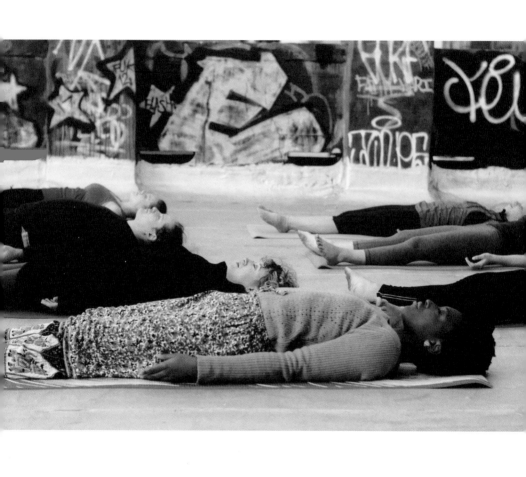

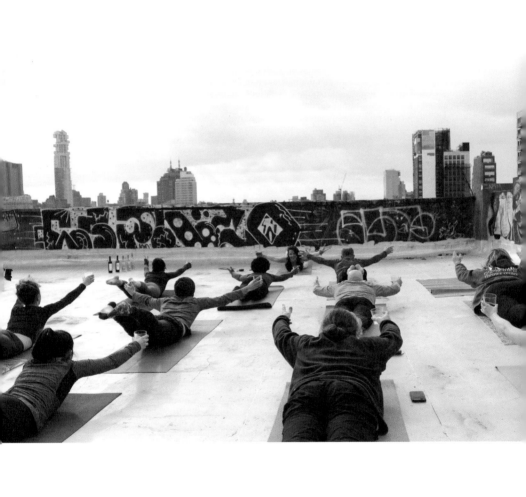

DRUNK YOGA® IS BETTER TOGETHER

I designed this class format specifically to exalt the feeling of levity that communal fun ignites.

Though, I have been told by many Drunk Yoga® fans that having a glass of wine before, or even while, they practice yoga on their own at home alone is their favorite way to yoga.

That said, since we're all about unity through community at Drunk Yoga®, here's a list of reasons why the art of blending wine with yoga is best enjoyed *among friends.*

1. When you lose your balance, you're surrounded by loving eyes to laugh at you. I mean laugh *with* you.

2. When you hold a pose that you've never been able to do before, you have someone right next to you always willing to give your glass a clink!

3. When you forget which pose you're supposed to do next, you can look at the person in front of you. And if it turns out that they, too, are doing the wrong pose, as least you'll both look ridiculous together, right?

4. *Somebody* has to take that Instagram photo of you sneaking a sip on your way into reverse warrior.

5. Fact: Happiness is better shared.

PARTNERS IN WINE

It's hard not to laugh at yourself when you're trying to balance a glass of wine in one hand while doing a yoga pose among a group of friends on the floor of a bar. (Or your kitchen, or your office . . .) One of the ways I like to teach people the art of "getting over themselves" is by gaining a new perspective through communicating with another. Or, in this particular exercise, through reaching your hands between your partner's legs (with consent). Let's explore . . .

In this Drunk Yoga® partner exercise, grab a partner (with consent) and a glass of wine. The exercise works best if you and your partner are about the same height, but it'll be much funnier if you're not. To begin, each of you must have a glass of wine in your right hand. Bend your knees as if you were about to squat into a tiny chair made for five-year-olds. Spread your legs about hips-width apart. Bring the glass of wine in between your legs from behind, far enough so your partner can grab hold of it with his/her left hand. Take hold of your partner's glass with your left hand. Repeat with the opposite hand.

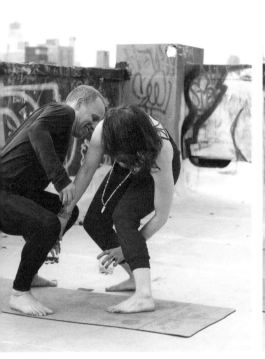
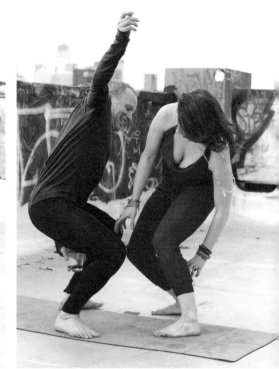
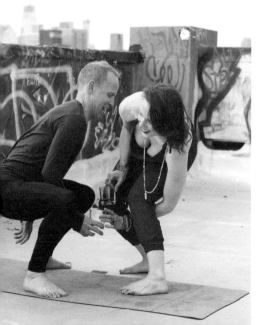
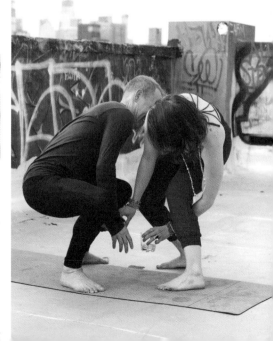

Bonus Drunk Yoga®: Partner Chair

Count backward from 10 with your partner in a language other than English (your language doesn't have to be the same as your partner's). And if you don't know how to count from 10 in another language by now, or aren't willing to learn, then, honestly, you probably deserve to sit here in discomfort for eternity.

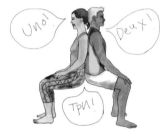

Bonus Drunk Yoga®: Partner Square

Choose a favorite song you both know and sing it together. If you can't think of a song you both know, choose your own song but sing them at the same time. Ex: "Twinkle, Twinkle Little Star" and "Don't Stop Believin'."

All right! That's done. Now should we all go get tattoos?

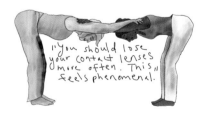

Drunk Yoga®: Syrah-can-asana

Essentially, sitting in a cross-legged position, known colloquially among five-year-olds as "crisscross applesauce."*

Sit up tall and relax your shoulders. Palms can either be faceup or facedown on your knees.

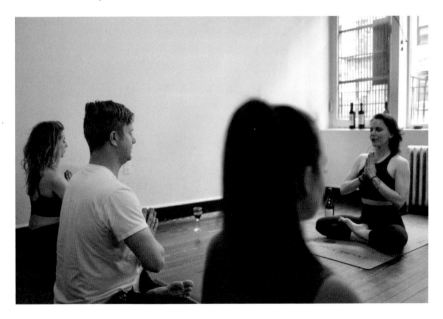

---

* No applesauce is to be consumed in the execution of this pose.

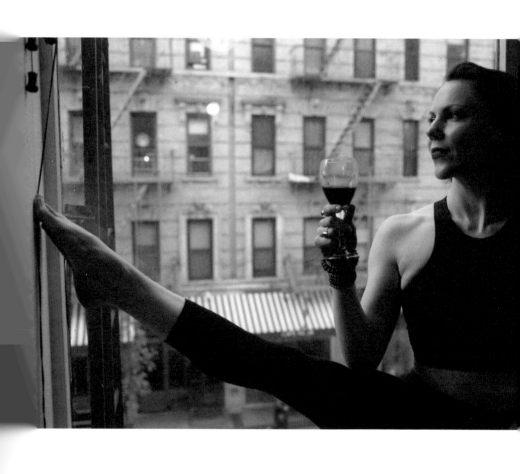

A̶F̶T̶E̶R̶W̶O̶R̶D̶ *BEFORE*-WORD

On my parents' refrigerator, which is located just outside of Madison, Wisconsin, there lives a postcard. And on that postcard is an illustration of a sheep standing on her hind legs behind a wooden fence. On that fence, there is a sign that reads, "BEWARE OF THE SHEEP." Underneath this sign is written a quote. And the quote reads . . . ahem: "Whenever you find yourself on the side of the majority, it's time to reform." —Mark Twain (Samuel Clemens, 1835–1910)

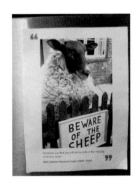

Chicken vs. egg. Which came first, the postcard on the fridge, or my natural inclination to go against the status quo? I think the latter, because I remember the comfort the postcard brought me when I read it for the first time in high school. It was self-assuring—that all of my weird aspirations to move to New York City and become an experimental performer/writer/philosopher/businesswoman were somehow in perfect "alignment." That I wasn't strange, I was just "reformational." And that all of the school lunches I spent eating with my band teacher in his office watching "how to" videos about the didgeridoo were 100 percent normal. So, too, were my Friday nights (and Saturday nights, for that matter, when I wasn't washing dishes at the local pub or refilling the salad bar at Pizza Hut) spent memorizing monologues from Lily Tomlin and Jane Wagner's *The Search for Signs of Intelligent Life in the Universe* and performing these monologues to my cats, parents, and anyone else who would listen (mostly just my cats and my parents).

In 2008, when it was time to apply to colleges, the woman who auditioned me for NYU asked, "Well, Elizabeth, is there anything else you'd like me to know?" I responded with a level of emotional intensity that only an eighteen-year-old aspiring drama major could get away with. I said that even though I didn't have much opportunity to act where I came from, and no professional experience to speak of (cue the violin), that I could, and *would*, work harder than any student she'd ever seen. She made a note on her clipboard, and it must have been favorable. Because, a few months later, I made my great Midwestern escape when I was offered a scholarship to New York University's Tisch School of the Arts for Acting. (Peace out, cats!)

And my *gosh* (that's what we say in Wisconsin) did I work hard. In classes, performances, internships, and at various day jobs—waitressing, bartending, catering, answering phones for the NYU housing office, and managing Stonestreet Studios, just to name a few. Understanding, even then, that having time for self-reflection was a privilege and not a right, I even worked hard at traveling and introspection. I worked so hard, in fact, that I was hospitalized twice for fatigue . . . (oops). If I were a robot, I'd have been wired with only one setting: overdrive. As a result, however, I managed to leverage every situation into a new work opportunity, out of necessity.

Fade to black, cut to 2014.

Now, equipped with an acting agent, a respectable résumé, a savings account, and a reserve of youthful vigor totally wasted on a twenty-four-year-old, I signed up for my yoga teacher training—something I'd looked forward to for several years, as I'd been casually dabbling in asana and meditation, albeit with fervent longing. I was eager to know what the yoga teachers know and also yearning for a day job that didn't involve refilling ketchup bottles.

So, here's where things got a bit rockier. I applied this same obsessive impulse to overachieve to my yoga practice. I exhausted myself as I strived to perform my asanas to perfection and win approval from my notoriously abusive teacher, taking two or three yoga class-es a day. In that year, despite the excessive *vinyasas*, meditation, and green juice, I grew extremely ill and fatigued because I was emotionally drained. This yoga wasn't working. I mean, listen, my body looked *great*—but my interior landscape was a mess. What had been a magical, mystical, and motivational refuge, yoga, to me, turned into a punishment. Yet another daily practice to remind me that I would never be whole—or at least would never meet the standards of perfection set by the elusive yoga elite required to achieve enlightenment.

Beyond burned out, I was dangerously sad. More accurately, I was knee-deep in a tumultuous quarter-life existential crisis. I cried most hours of every day, unable to get out of bed. Life was inherently meaningless, I thought. And if everything is only temporary, then what's the f*cking point? I felt it to my core—the invisible, karmic soul kind of core—that reality as I knew it was an illusion, and I didn't know how to cope. (Ugh, thanks a *lot*, yoga.)

Not one for moping, I bought a one-way ticket to India and back-packed by myself across the country for several months, desper-ately seeking answers to the *biggest* questions. "If everything is divinely orchestrated, then what is 'choice,' and where do my thoughts come from? Or, if 'free will' is a thing, then who am *I* to choose my path?" I went to all the yoga courses, the tantra medita-tions, the Satsangs with Mooji, Prem Baba, and this radical British Buddhist nun whose name I really wish I remembered. I even did a ten-day silent Vipassana meditation retreat outside of a Buddhist temple in Dharamsala. My *gosh* was I seeking. I spent hours each morning floating in the Arabian Sea, wondering, "Who am I? How did Earth get here? What *makes* the thoughts that are asking these questions, and how could they belong to me if I am no one?"

After about four months, my intestines were ripe with parasites, and I was thoroughly sleep deprived. So I flew to Thailand to decompress. Almost as soon as I arrived on the island of Koh Tao, however (plot twist!), I fell through a roof and severely injured my back (long story).

"Why were you on the roof, Eli?" asks everyone who hears this story. "Don't ask," I respond to everyone who asks me that question, which is everyone who hears this story. "It doesn't matter," I add with a pitiful sigh, to draw out suspense and capitalize on the sympathy I get from my listeners who never fail to look confused whenever they hear this story.

At this point, of course, I thought my relationship with yoga was over for good.

But thanks to the kindness of strangers who, subsequently, became good friends (and by "strangers," I mean my scuba diving instructor whose roof I'd just destroyed), and the neighbor's fortuitous extra stash of powerful painkillers (again, don't ask), I was able to stand up after about a week of immobility and hobble my way to a local juice bar.

So, there I was, sitting at this juice bar feeling pretty sorry for myself, when along came a man who was the spitting image of *The Simpsons'* "Comic Book Guy" character, sans shirt and shoes. He sat down on the juice bar stool next to mine, and he ordered a coconut and wheat grass shot. With a wide grin and a lisp, he asked the skinny, blond twenty-year-old who was juice-tending behind the bar, "So, Becky, what do you want to talk about today?" Without looking up from her phone, Becky responded (mid gum-chew), "Um, I don't care." Unfazed by her apathy, Comic Book Guy smiled again and said, "How about the illusion of time?" Still swiping on Instagram, Becky unenthusiastically responded, "Um, sure."

My ears, however, perked up higher than the painkillers made me feel when I heard his preferred topic of conversation. Momentarily, climbing out of my pool of self-pity, I said to the guy,

"Actually, um, hi, I'm Eli, and I'd love to talk about the illusion of time."

"Great!" he exclaimed, "Well, the concept of time is—"

I interrupted, "Actually, can I ask you a question?"

"Sure!" (Remember he had a lisp so just make sure you hear that word in your mind with a lisp.)

"Is everything in life divinely orchestrated? And if so, how do you define 'free will'?"

In the timeless minutes that followed (because minutes are an illusion, remember), the literal backbreaking weight of existential dread I'd been carrying finally started to evaporate. Because Comic Book Guy was actually a quantum physicist from the United States, currently living in Thailand and working with a team of other scientists on a cure for AIDS. Meanwhile, he was also quite spiritual, and he explained to me this:

The respective concepts of "divine orchestration" and "free will" both simultaneously exist and do not exist, because they are both constructs of the grasping human mind. "The eye can't see the eye," and it's not meant to. A piece of the whole will never be able to fathom the greatness of what it comprises. In other words, it is not our job, nor our right, as human beings to understand whether our fates are preordered, and if everything is "meant to be," or if we are indeed the maker of our own destinies. What seekers must accept is that there are infinite forces of the universe beyond our capacity to see that are perpetually at work, making every interaction, thought, and "decision" not only possible, but inevitable.

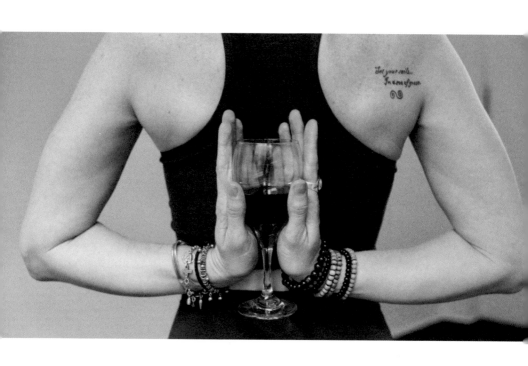

From this conversation, I gleaned that our perceived "free will," or rather, our choices, are divine, simply because we make them.

Unashamed tears of cosmic relief streamed down my cheeks as I then asked Comic Book Scientist Guy, "Okay. Awesome. That's great. That clears up a lot for me, thanks. But listen, as soon as my back is healed, I have to go back to New York City, and I have to decide if I'm going to be an actress or a yoga teacher. How do I make this choice if I am an illusion and all my 'choices' are divine?" And he paused and then answered deliberately and profoundly, "Just set your sails in a sea of grace, and . . ."

. . . And I can't friggin' remember what he said after that, but whatever, it's fine. The first part was good enough.

Like any good hippie-solo-backpacker, I got this phrase tattooed on my back—specifically atop the ribs that I'd just cracked—in a small Thai tattoo parlor by a squatting barefoot Thai man using a sharp bamboo stick while smoking a cigarette. And after about seven weeks of restless back healing on Koh Tao, I was finally ready to pack my things and begin my next journey: returning to New York City to deal with #adulting.

Fatefully, upon my return to New York, I discovered Katonah Yoga, created by Nevine Michaan, which not only helped me to heal from my back injury, but was a philosophical game changer. Through her restorative Hatha practice, beautifully interwoven with Taoist theory and sacred geometry, she taught me that the universe has no personal investment in my happiness. (Gasp!)

The universe will continue to run by its own laws, regardless of my feelings about it. The universe does not care if I am happy or healthy—only I do. And because I am the only being personally invested in the quality of my life, it is up to me to hone ways of achieving my own sense of joy, working with the laws of the nature—not in spite of them.

Through an extremely progressive, esoteric yoga practice, she taught me that "everything you see is true, but so is everything you don't see. So, the question is not 'is this true, or is that true?' The question you should ask yourself is 'Why am I seeing this truth instead of that truth?'"

That's all I needed.

Now I knew that both "darkness" and "light" (and all that they entail) were equally true and "untrue," depending on how I told the story; that is to say, the story that "life is meaningless" is just as valid as the story that "my life is full of purpose." So I decided then that I would equip myself with more tools that would enable me to choose which story I'd like to have as *my* experience. I quickly redirected my focus to living an empowered life and subsequently learned about creating healthy esoteric boundaries through cultivating my own techniques for personal joy. I crawled out of my figurative black pit of existential (yogic) dread, and built a new (happy) life from scratch. And, between you and me, it is a life that I'm quite proud of . . . mostly because—you guessed it—I worked really, really hard for it.

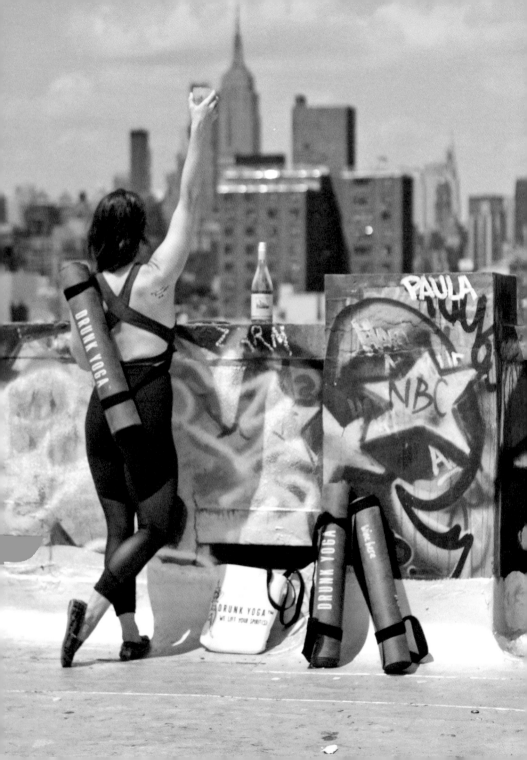